Helping kids have a healthy relationship with sex and their bodies starts when they're young. But as a parent sometimes I don't know what to say or how to say it! In this book, Dr. Laura Hancock and Dr. Karen Rayne offer an informative, practical, and readable guide to navigating this tricky area. I learned a lot from this book and feel empowered to have better conversations with my children.

—**DEBBIE SORENSEN, PhD,** COHOST OF *PSYCHOLOGISTS OFF THE CLOCK* PODCAST AND AUTHOR OF *ACT FOR BURNOUT* AND *ACT DAILY JOURNAL*

Sex Ed for the Stroller Set is a precious gift to families, children, and educators everywhere. In a culture where "sex ed" for young children is so often reduced to the notion of "The Talk," Hancock and Rayne brilliantly capture—page by page by page—the countless ways that supporting healthy sexual development resides in the daily living experiences within families and schools and as an integral part of a child's ongoing physical, social, emotional, and intellectual development.

—**DEBORAH M. ROFFMAN, MS, CSE, CFLE,** HUMAN SEXUALITY EDUCATOR, AUTHOR, AND CONSULTANT

T0277520

Those of us who've worked in the sexuality field have long observed that young people and adults who have a childhood with thoughtful and comfortable bodies, relationships, sex and boundaries information, and parenting usually have much better outcomes than those who don't. Positive parenting in this department is something we know tends to result in more fulfilling and comfortable sexual lives, healthier and more beneficial relationships, better body image and boundaries, and real ownership and understanding of one's own sexual agency, autonomy, and identity.

Many parents and caregivers want to provide all of this and more for children, but they don't know how, or they feel so overwhelmed or intimidated that they freeze up even trying to start. Enter *Sex Ed for the Stroller Set* and the incredible wealth of information and empathetic coaching Karen and Laura provide within its pages. *Sex Ed for the Stroller Set* is holistic and rich while also being very easy to read and digest. You'll find information about childhood sexual development by stages and sexuality, self-awareness help for yourself, and other vital basics like anatomy, gender, orientation, boundaries, and abuse prevention and awareness, presented in practical, useful, and actionable ways. I feel certain every reader of this book will feel more knowledgeable, confident, and comfortable as a parent sex educator than they imagined they could before they found it.

–HEATHER CORINNA, AUTHOR AND FOUNDER OF SCARLETEEN

sex ed
FOR THE
stroller set

sex ed
FOR THE
stroller set

HOW TO HAVE
HONEST CONVERSATIONS
WITH YOUNG CHILDREN

laura hancock, phd
& karen rayne, phd

 AMERICAN PSYCHOLOGICAL ASSOCIATION

Published by
APA LifeTools
750 First Street, NE
Washington, DC 20002
https://www.apa.org

Order Department
https://www.apa.org/pubs/books
order@apa.org

Typeset in Sabon by Circle Graphics, Inc., Reisterstown, MD

Printer: Sheridan Books, Chelsea, MI
Cover Designer: Mark Karis

Library of Congress Cataloging-in-Publication Data

Names: Hancock, Laura, author. | Rayne, Karen, author.
Title: Sex ed for the stroller set : how to have honest conversations with
   young children / by Laura Hancock and Karen Rayne.
Description: Washington, DC : American Psychological Association, [2023] |
   Includes bibliographical references and index.
Identifiers: LCCN 2023006321 (print) | LCCN 2023006322 (ebook) |
   ISBN 9781433838439 (paperback) | ISBN 9781433838446 (ebook)
Subjects: LCSH: Sex instruction for children. | Children and sex. |
   Parenting. | BISAC: FAMILY & RELATIONSHIPS / Parenting / General |
   EDUCATION / Teaching / Subjects / Health & Sexuality
Classification: LCC HQ57 .H356 2023 (print) | LCC HQ57 (ebook) |
   DDC 649/.65--dc23/eng/20230413
LC record available at https://lccn.loc.gov/2023006321
LC ebook record available at https://lccn.loc.gov/2023006322

https://doi.org/10.1037/0000368-000

Printed in the United States of America

10 9 8 7 6 5 4 3 2 1

CONTENTS

sex ed

FOR THE

stroller set

Introduction:
Sex Ed Begins at Birth

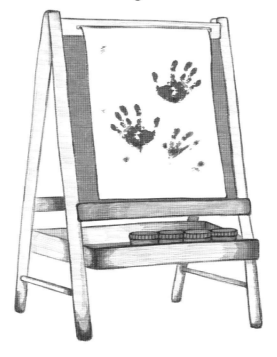

Laura, one of the coauthors of this book, walked into her friend Jen's[1] house one hot Texas afternoon and was excited to greet two of her favorite kids. This particular afternoon, Mia, now 3 years old, and Logan, age 5 years, were sitting around in their underwear, too busy playing to say hello. They were immersed in their game of

[1]To protect people's privacy, we have changed the names of all individuals included in our stories.

doctor and patient. Logan was playing the role of doctor. He had removed the round end of a toy stethoscope. With the earpieces snugly around his leg, he was holding the end of the stethoscope hose inside the back of Mia's underwear and "removing her farts." Each time Mia made a farting sound, they would both burst into laughter. Laura noticed, however, that Jen was not laughing. She wasn't panicking, but Laura could see she was uncomfortable, rolling her eyes and smiling sheepishly. She had grown up in a home in which this kind of play would not have been acceptable. Jen knew she wanted to raise her children differently from the way she had been raised. She wanted to be the kind of parent who talked openly with her kids about bodies, bodily functions, privacy, and all the other sexuality topics she could name. And yet, at a moment like this, she didn't know quite what to do. Should she let them play in this way? Should she stop them? How should she stop them? What should she say?

This "removing the farts" episode began a conversation between Jen and Laura. They started to talk about the many situations in which Jen wasn't quite sure what to do. A lot of parents come to both of us—Laura and Karen—with similar questions and uncertainty. At what age should they stop bathing with their child? What can they say when their child asks how the new baby got into Mommy's tummy? What is the best way to respond when their child is playing with their genitals while sitting on the sofa? In this book, we answer these questions (and more), and we help you to understand and respond to situations like these. We also help you to feel more confident and comfortable as we work our way toward becoming a more unshockable, approachable, go-to parent—the kind of parent kids want to talk with when they have questions or concerns about sexuality.

When it comes to teaching kids about sexuality, some educators recommend a more cautionary approach. In this reactive approach, parents do not bring up topics about sexuality themselves, but they do answer children's questions and react appropriately to situations that occur. If a child asks a question, people with this approach recommend that parents make sure to fully clarify the question and then address only the question asked. The approach we take is proactive—one in which parents intentionally teach their child about sexuality, the same way we would teach them about other topics. We don't wait for a child to ask what color something is or how to say the alphabet, nor do we wait for them to ask about the safest way to cross the street. We teach children all kinds of things about nature, like how plants grow or how to find worms. The same should be true for teaching kids about sexuality. We shouldn't wait for them to ask. Some kids are really curious and ask a lot of questions. Other children are less verbal or ask fewer questions, but they are often just as curious and always need just as much information as children who ask lots of questions. We believe that all children deserve to know information that will help to keep them healthy and safe.

The aim of this book is to equip you to create a strong foundation of sexual health in your child, rather than just handle a particular situation. We give you the tools you need to proactively teach your child about topics that will help them grow into adults with healthy, fulfilling, and pleasurable sex lives and relationships.

This book is intended to help you to

- understand sexuality and what sexual health comprises,
- learn what behaviors and topics are appropriate and essential during early childhood,
- learn tools to teach your child what they need to know about sexuality,
- know what to teach your child to keep them safer from sexual abuse,
- handle the surprising situations and questions you get from your child,

- envision the healthy sexuality you want for your child now and in the future,
- practice techniques for calming your anxiety and feeling confident when talking about sexual topics, and
- become a go-to parent/caregiver and establish a lifelong dialogue with your child about topics that are essential to their well-being.

WHY IS IT HELPFUL TO START TEACHING ABOUT SEXUALITY AT SUCH YOUNG AGES?

This book is for you if you are a parent, caregiver, teacher, or anyone else working with children in *early childhood*, which is defined as the years from birth through age 6 years. For simplicity, we refer to caregivers as "parents" throughout this book. It is important to note, however, that this book is meant for anyone caring for a young child or children.

You may wonder why you should start teaching your child about sexual health from such an early age. Here are some of the most important reasons.

You Are Already Teaching Your Child About Sexuality

Sexuality is about so much more than sex. Sexuality is also about appreciating your own body and keeping it healthy. It's about requiring others to respect you and your boundaries. It's about healthy relationships and being aware of your feelings. Through your behaviors, attitudes, feelings, and words, your child is learning about all these topics already. This book strives to help you to make informed decisions about what and how you teach about sexuality. *In this way, you can be conscious of messages you are sending your child, rather than teaching them blindly.*

They Want to Know

Children are naturally curious and eager to soak up information about the world around them. Just as they are fascinated by construction vehicles, bugs, cleaning, or anything else, they are intensely curious about bodies and relationships. This is a wonderful opportunity for us parents to teach them about many aspects of sexuality. *By starting early, we can take advantage of their curiosity and their lack of self-consciousness.*

By Starting Now, You Get to Practice Having Sexuality-Related Conversations

For many parents, thinking or talking about sexuality and bodies can provoke anxiety. For others, they feel comfortable with the topic, but talking with their kids about it just doesn't feel natural. Perhaps they don't know what to say, or they don't know what to do with all the feelings that come up. Just imagine, however, that your child is now a preteen or teenager. Now, a new set of sexual health topics is emerging in their life. They are entering puberty. They are having more sexual feelings. They are hearing things at school. They are exposed to more media. *If you have already had ongoing conversations with your child about sexuality, you will have had years of practice navigating sexuality-related topics with them before the stakes are higher.* Your child will already have a solid foundation of information from which they can process new experiences. And they will have practice coming to *you* when they need help and have questions.

Knowledge Is Protection

Childhood sexual abuse cannot always be prevented, and it is *never* the fault of the child. *Nevertheless, there are things we can do to lower the risk of abuse.* One of those things is to give children accurate language for sexual topics. This protects children by making predators less likely to engage with them because the child clearly has an adult they are able to talk with about sexuality. Creating open lines of communication between you and your child increases the chance that you will find out if something inappropriate does happen to them. Without instilling fear, you can teach your child to expect their boundaries to be respected and to respect the boundaries of others through all stages of life.

You Are Your Young Child's Best Sex Ed Teacher

As a parent or primary caregiver, you are the person best suited to teach your young child about these topics. Early on, your child will get all their information from a small number of people, including you and other primary caregivers. They will develop a deep level of trust and connection with you. This is the time to pour in all the good feelings, values, and information you want them to have. As your child gets older, their world will expand, they will naturally gain broader influences in their life, and they will remain curious. Older kids will inevitably have a broader access to information about sexuality through the internet, other media, and their peers. Not all this exposure will be helpful, healthy, or accurate. If you have been educating them and giving them accurate resources, your child will be more equipped to discern fact from fiction and get answers to their questions in appropriate ways. One of the best ways your child can get accurate information is from you. When you show your child early on that you answer their questions without anger, shame, or judgment and that you talk about hard topics, you become the kind of parent whom they can trust with their questions.

Sexual Health Is Fundamental to Your Child's Well-Being

As parents, we have an instinctive urge to help our child be happy and fulfilled, and we work really hard to give our child the best start in life that we can. *Sexual health is essential to overall health.* Helping your child develop healthy sexuality from their earliest years is one of the greatest gifts you can give your child.

ABOUT THE AUTHORS

Laura and Karen each started teaching about sexual health in different ways.

Laura

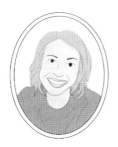

Laura had a meandering route to her role in sexual health education. She grew up outside Chicago with a father who worked in graphic design and mother who was a nurse. Along with her two siblings, she was encouraged to foster her talents in both art and science, and in 1997, she earned her bachelor of fine arts degree from Washington University in St. Louis. Along with her desire to explore the world through art, Laura had always been fascinated by the intersection between human biology and behavior, and she completed a second major in physical anthropology while earning her bachelor's degree. Eventually, she decided to pursue a graduate degree at The University of Texas at Austin, where she studied biological anthropology and psychology. Her research, which took her to various field sites in places such as Costa Rica and Madagascar, focused on understanding human evolution and behavior through the study of the anatomy, biology, and behavior of nonhuman primates (i.e., apes, monkeys, and lemurs). During her graduate career, she was asked to give a guest lecture for a class on primate biology for which she chose to include a lot of information about human reproductive biology. Following the lecture, a student approached her and said, "Thank you for teaching that class. I never knew about any of that stuff." That moment stuck with her.

After earning her doctoral degree in anthropology in 2009, Laura wanted to apply her academic interests and her love of teaching and writing to something new. She shifted her focus to helping young people understand their own body and biology, feel good about themselves, and make healthy decisions. In 2012, Laura became certified to teach kids aged 5 to 19 years about sexual health. Throughout her training in sexual health education, she realized that most of the sexuality topics young people learn about are already important before children enter elementary school. But there was a catch: Although parents of young children had encountered situations in which they wanted to teach their child about sexuality, it was rare that they felt confident about what was appropriate or what to do. Thus, Laura created a unique, new curriculum teaching parents and other caregivers how to educate young children about healthy sexuality.

Laura now lives in Amsterdam, the Netherlands, with her husband and daughter. There, she likes to walk in nature, study Dutch, see art, make art, read, and enjoy their bikecentric city.

Karen

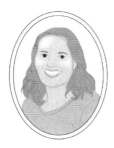

Karen is originally from Texas and has felt called to work with teenagers since she was a teenager. She originally set out to be a high school English teacher but quickly realized that the topic wasn't the right match for her teaching career. After nevertheless earning her bachelor of arts degree in English and secondary education, Karen went back to school to get her master of arts degree and doctoral degree in educational psychology. In her last semester of grad school, the same month as she was defending her dissertation and still not sure what she would do professionally when she graduated, Karen was asked to provide sex education for a friend and her teenage daughter who had experienced a pregnancy scare. Karen dove in, fell in love with the content, and hasn't looked back since! In the subsequent 20 years, Karen's focus has expanded from teenagers to a lifespan approach to sexuality education. She has worked at and written for universities, nonprofits, United Nations affiliates, and with individuals all around the world.

OTHER VOICES

Throughout this book you will also hear from other parents. In an effort to provide you with real-life parenting examples from a diverse group of caregivers, we sent out requests via social media to look for parents who would be willing to write down some of their stories. The seven contributors who got in touch with us are all parents or coparents. Some are friends and colleagues, and others we have never met. From both the United States and the Netherlands, these contributors offer some interesting insights into the similarities and differences between the two cultures.

Like these seven contributors, every parent we have talked with has a story (or many!) about the sexuality questions or situations they have encountered with their child. Most parents have been taken by surprise at some point by their child's sexuality questions or behavior. We view these surprises as a fun and challenging part of the parenting journey that keeps us on our toes.

We have included one last group of contributors in this book. At the end of Chapter 10, you can read success stories from three families in which the parents have made a concerted effort to talk openly and honestly with their children about sexuality from the beginning. You will also get to hear from grown children in these families. These testimonials illustrate what we can look forward to in the future: Adult children who feel free to talk with us parents about their questions and experiences, who feel pride and agency over their own sexuality, and who have been supported with knowledge rather than hindered by shame.

ABOUT THIS BOOK

This book is separated into two parts. Part I, What You Need to Know First, gives you background information to prepare you for teaching your child and includes these chapters:

- Chapter 1 is an introduction to understanding sexuality from a holistic perspective.
- Chapter 2 helps you to prepare by getting to know yourself a bit better. This chapter on self-awareness is an important one because regulating your emotions is one of the key components to teaching your child about sexuality without shame.
- In Chapters 3 and 4, we get you up to speed with concepts and terms related to gender identity, sexual orientation, and reproductive anatomy and physiology.
- Chapter 5 is dedicated to one of the most pressing issues around sexual health: understanding, preventing, and responding to child sexual abuse.

Part II of the book, The Ages and Stages of Teaching Sexual Health During Early Childhood, is dedicated to giving you all the practical information you need to know to teach your young child about healthy sexuality. This part consists of these chapters:

- Chapters 6, 7, and 8 discuss the three age groups in early childhood—infancy, toddlerhood, and kindergarten—in which we let you know *how* kids are learning, *what* they are learning about sexuality, and how *you* can teach them.

- Chapter 9 is dedicated to responding to surprising questions and situations.
- Chapter 10, the last chapter, is about some of the things you can expect in later years.

As you read the stories and chapters in this book, we hope you'll recognize your own hopes and struggles. Know that you are not alone on this journey.

1

What You Need to Know First

1ST

INTRODUCTION: WHAT YOU NEED TO KNOW FIRST

Before we offer you specific tools for teaching about sexual health, we want to establish a collective, solid foundation of knowledge. To be effective while teaching our children about sexual health, we first need two kinds of knowledge: (a) fundamental concepts and terms around sexuality and (b) self-knowledge. Our hope is that once equipped with this information, you will feel more confident and prepared to provide your child with accurate and honest knowledge about sexuality.

This part of the book provides important material about sexuality that you can use to teach your child. It is not, however, intended as a teaching aid to show or read to your child. (See the resources for that in Part II of the book.) If a lot of this material is new to you, you are not alone. Many of us go through life without ever having any formal sexuality education. The information included here covers the basic content you need for teaching your child during early childhood (infancy through age 6 years). As your child gets older, you will have the opportunity to read other books about the topics they need to know next.

Part I comprises five chapters:

- Chapter 1. What Is Sexuality?
- Chapter 2. Parental Self-Awareness: History, Feelings, and Values

- Chapter 3. Reproductive Anatomy and Physiology
- Chapter 4. Gender and Sexual Orientation
- Chapter 5. Child Sexual Abuse: Prevention and Response

Even if you are well-versed in these topics, we recommend you read through them so that we share a common terminology throughout the rest of the book.

Chapter 1
What Is Sexuality?

We are sexual beings from the time we are born. Indeed, infants are particularly sensual; they are rooted in physicality, experiencing the world through their senses. As infants grow, and especially into toddlerhood, the ways in which children are sexual become more apparent. Toddlers are famous (or perhaps infamous) for doing sexual things that are awkward or embarrassing for us grown-ups. Without the boundaries and inhibitions that they will eventually develop, they play with their genitals in public or loudly ask, "Why do you have nipples if you don't have boobs to feed the baby?" Then, as young children enter school, they encounter a new set of social circumstances in which curiosity about everything from marriage to genitals gets discussed among their wizened peer group. Because people are sexual from the beginning, parents are faced with various aspects of their child's sexuality before puberty is even on the horizon.

In Part II of this book, we discuss the developmentally appropriate behaviors of infants, toddlers, and kindergartners in more detail, and you'll get to read numerous examples of the things kids say and do and ideas for how to respond. For now, however, we'd like to consider what sexuality is from a more theoretical perspective. We first want to help you appreciate the ways in which sexuality reaches into almost every aspect of our lives, some of which may not be obvious at first. The term *sexuality* encompasses the topics of anatomy and physiology of reproduction, attraction, emotional and physical intimacy, eroticism, gender identity, gender roles, physical health, pleasure, relationships, sexual orientation, and many more. Sexuality is a complex interplay of all these and other facets to differing degrees at any given time.

Your child has their own individual sexuality. Their sexuality will constantly form and shift over their lifetime, it will be influenced by countless internal and external dynamics, and it will change as their body changes. It will be influenced by their personality, what they encounter in their social groups, what they see in the media, and even by current laws and medicine. During early childhood, *your* behaviors and attitudes will have the greatest influence. And yet, their sexuality is still their own. It is your job as a parent to remain curious about who your child is and who they are becoming, to help them understand and navigate their sexuality and to support them in their journey.

Comprehending the complexity of sexuality can help you to understand yourself and your child better. Because it is so complex and far reaching, we have two different ways for you to consider sexuality as a holistic concept. The first model is called the *four perspectives* model of sexuality and the second is the *sexualitree*.

THE FOUR PERSPECTIVES MODEL OF SEXUALITY

This framework provides insight into sexuality by discussing it from four perspectives, all of which are integrated: physical, emotional, cognitive, and social.

Physical

Healthy sexuality from a physical perspective means a person is safe from abuse and takes measures to be free from illness and to promote physical health. It means they are free to experience erotic pleasure and that their need for *non*erotic touch is also getting met.

Questions to consider for raising young children. In what ways can you teach your child to care for their body and keep it healthy? How can you fulfill your child's need for nonerotic affection? How can you show how important and wonderful affection is and also model how to express and maintain clear boundaries? What do you teach your child about safety, their erotic desires, and the need for pleasure?

Emotional

Healthy sexuality from an emotional perspective is the ability to be in touch with one's desires, needs, and feelings. It is the capacity for love, trust, vulnerability, and attachment. It is the ability to engage in connected, fulfilling, and lasting relationships. The emotional component of sexuality can be very much entwined with the physical aspect. Skin-to-skin contact is one of the first ways we fulfill the emotional needs of our child. Infants learn love, trust, and attachment through touch. When we give and receive physical affection, our brains produce hormones like oxytocin, which produces feelings of love and connection.

Questions to consider for raising young children. How can you teach your child about emotions? How can you help your child to be attuned to their own emotions while behaving in ways that are age appropriate? How can you avoid instilling feelings of shame or insecurity around sexuality?

Cognitive

From a cognitive perspective, sexuality relates to a person's thoughts, opinions, attitudes, self-awareness, and how they perceive themselves and their identity. This aspect of sexuality includes all the factual information you will teach your child, and it is how your child will come to think about sexuality and about themselves. Healthy sexuality from a cognitive perspective includes a healthy body image and self-love. One's cognitive perspective is closely tied to their feelings about themselves and others.

Questions to consider for raising young children. How can you teach your child factual information about sexuality in age-appropriate ways? How can you encourage self-love, self-esteem, and self-acceptance? How can you help your child explore and understand their own identity?

Social

The social aspect of sexuality relates to all the different messages we get from the world around us. These messages come from family, school friends, teachers, faith groups, and the culture in which we live. Different people and groups of people have various social norms when it comes to sexuality. Many of these messages become part of who we are without any conscious thought on our part. As children grow older, however, they will take more opportunities to decide which messages they will integrate into their own value system.

Questions to consider for raising young children. What are the most important messages and values you want to teach your child? How do we, as a society, teach about values? How do we discuss the different and sometimes conflicting messages in the world around us?

None of these four perspectives on sexuality—physical, emotional, cognitive, or social—is mutually exclusive; there is overlap among all of them. A good example of this overlap is when we teach about boundaries. Children need to learn skills to set healthy boundaries within all four of these categories of sexuality. For instance, we set physical boundaries with others by communicating how we agree to be touched. We set emotional boundaries by not taking on, or feeling responsible for, another person's feelings. We set cognitive boundaries when we separate our own identity from those of others and maintain a coherent sense of self without being overly influenced by others' opinions. In the social aspect of sexuality, we experience all the different cultural norms for boundaries. Moreover, one of the important ways we know that our physical or cognitive boundaries are being pushed is by awareness of how we feel emotionally. Nervousness, anxiety, or worry can all be indicators that we need to establish a new boundary with someone. Thus, this one concept of boundary setting is an important part of all aspects of sexuality.

Each aspect of sexuality also influences the other aspects (see the figure on the four perspectives model of sexuality). Our hormones (physical) can affect how we feel (emotions). Our religion or moral context (social) can affect how we view ourselves and our own decisions (cognitive). For examples, see the table that follows. One of the most exciting jobs as a parent is the opportunity to teach your child how to integrate all these aspects of themselves. You can help them learn from an early age how to pay attention to what their body is telling them and how to think about their feelings.

Examples of Sexuality From Each of the Four Perspectives

Physical	Emotional	Cognitive	Social
Reproductive anatomy and physiology	Intimacy	Identity	Values
	Attachment	Attitudes	Family
Need for touch	Love	Body image	Religion
Pleasure	Empathy	Self-awareness	Culture
Physical health	Vulnerability	Self-love	Medicine
Boundaries	Trust	Self-esteem	Politics
			History

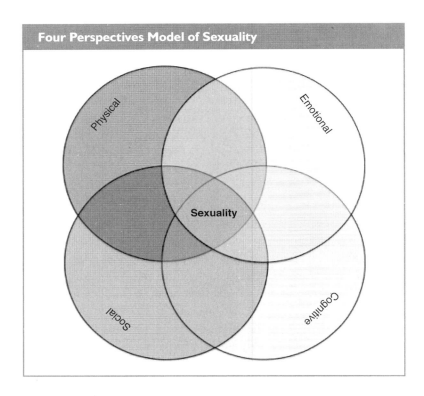

THE SEXUALITREE

Another way to conceptualize the extent of what sexuality includes is by considering the sexualitree (see the figure). This model invites us to consider the ways that many different elements related to sexuality (including all of the examples listed earlier and more) influence us at the cultural, relational, and intimate levels.

The cultural level includes the broad messaging and influences of the media; government; religious institutions; language; and other large-scale, culture-wide influences. These messages begin when a person is very young and have substantial influences on the ways

The Sexualitree

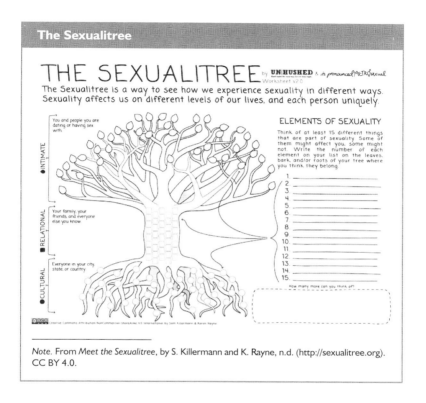

THE SEXUALITREE by **UNHUSHED** *(it's pronounced METROsexual)*
Worksheet v2.0

The Sexualitree is a way to see how we experience sexuality in different ways. Sexuality affects us on different levels of our lives, and each person uniquely.

You and people you are dating or having sex with

● INTIMATE

Your family, your friends, and everyone else you know

● RELATIONAL

Everyone in your city, state, or country

● CULTURAL

ELEMENTS OF SEXUALITY

Think of at least 15 different things that are part of sexuality. Some of them might affect you. Some might not. Write the number of each element on your list on the leaves, bark, and/or roots of your tree where you think they belong.

1 _____
2 _____
3 _____
4 _____
5 _____
6 _____
7 _____
8 _____
9 _____
10 _____
11 _____
12 _____
13 _____
14 _____
15 _____

How many more can you think of?

Note. From *Meet the Sexualitree*, by S. Killermann and K. Rayne, n.d. (http://sexualitree.org). CC BY 4.0.

that they think and move through the world. These messages take longer to change than at the other two levels and are often fundamental to people's relational and individual experiences.

The relational level includes the messages people get from their family and friends and others whom they actually know. These messages include the kinds of things you tell your child directly, the things that other caregivers tell them, and eventually the things that their friends and peers tell them.

The intimate level is often more about experiences than it is about messages. These experiences include, for young children,

25

whether and how they play doctor with their friends, whether their house is one where people are nude or always clothed, how they experience gender, and other personally relevant experiences.

The ways that each of these elements influence a person ultimately form their own unique sexualitree. (For more information on this model, you can visit http://sexualitree.org/.)

Frameworks and models are designed to give people the most effective perspective on the topic at hand. If you have found these conceptualizations of sexuality useful in expanding your understanding of sexuality, they have done their job! However, they are always imperfect. If you find yourself feeling that these explanations of sexuality do not fully describe your own experiences, you are seeing where they can fall short. If this is your experience, we invite you to create your own model or perspective of the vast experience that is human sexuality! More work in this area is always warranted and exciting.

SUMMARY

- People are sexual throughout our lives, beginning in infancy. Moreover, sexuality is integrated into almost every aspect of our lives.
- Here we want to help you expand your understanding of sexuality from a more theoretical perspective before we get into all the practical information in Part II. To do this, we offer two models, or two different ways of conceptualizing sexuality: the four perspectives model of sexuality and the sexualitree. These models are not perfect, but they are intended to help you think about a topic that is quite complex.
- As you consider these models, you can think about how they apply to your own sexuality and that of your child.

RESOURCES FOR PARENTS

- *How to Understand Your Sexuality: A Practical Guide for Exploring Who You Are* by Meg-John Barker and Alex Iantaffi (Jessica Kingsley Publishers)
- *Human Sexuality: Diversity in Contemporary Society* (10th ed.) by William L. Yarber and Barbara W. Sayad (McGraw Hill Education)
- *Meet the Sexualitree*: http://sexualitree.org/
- *The Right to Sex: Feminism in the Twenty-First Century* by Amia Srinivasan (Farrar, Straus and Giroux)

Chapter 2
Parental Self-Awareness:
History, Feelings, and Values

Kim, a mother Laura knows, had parents whose views about sexuality differed significantly from the environment in which she had been raised. Kim's parents were willing to discuss sexual topics to some degree, but they had a lot of narrow opinions about sexual feelings and behavior. They also had a lot of rules they wanted her to follow. Conversely, the community in which they lived was very open about sexuality, but some of the kids were engaging in unhealthy sexual behaviors.

Now, a parent herself, Kim found that she wanted to have open discussions about sexuality with her child, but she had no model for what to say. She didn't want to have discussions like she'd had with her parents: those laden with judgment. At the same time, she worried that her child would engage in the kind of sexual behaviors she had seen in her peers. How could she encourage healthy behaviors without resorting to judgment and rules? Laura suggested focusing on factual, age-appropriate information and family values instead of rules. First, however, Kim was encouraged to spend time writing about and discussing her history, her fears, and what she wanted for her child in the future. Although her concerns haven't disappeared, she has found she is now able to discuss sexual topics with her child with a greater sense of tranquility and confidence.

If you feel anxious about talking openly about sexuality with your child, you're not alone. The idea of talking with their kids about sexual topics makes many parents nervous. We understand. We can tell you from personal experience and from the experiences of other parents that the more you do it, the more comfortable the process will become. It takes practice. Moreover, when parents *have* talked with their kids about the topics in this book, even topics that were difficult for them, they tell us that they were glad they did. So, if you're feeling squeamish, think about all the reasons to talk about sexuality that we listed in the introduction and how much you want to promote your child's health and safety. It's worth it.

SEX EDUCATION IN OUR FAMILY OF ORIGIN

Sexuality can be a rewarding, awkward, funny, fun, and confusing topic. When interacting with your child, we want your responses and the messages you convey to be the ones that are best for them. Sometimes, however, a parent's unresolved history and feelings can get in the way. It's normal for old, unconscious habits and beliefs to surface when you begin to observe, respond to, and teach your child about different sexuality topics. For example, if we are nervous about using correct terminology for reproductive anatomy, we might inadvertently communicate that genitals are something that really shouldn't be talked about. If we have grown up in an environment in which sexual pleasure wasn't supposed to be expressed until adulthood, we might unwittingly shame our child when we see them explore their body. If we were sexually abused, we might be hypervigilant when it comes to our child and teach them that they have much to fear rather than that they have support and resources available if someone harms them.

Each of us has had our own experiences learning about sex and sexuality. Some of us grew up in a family that was open about sexuality and that viewed sexuality as a normal part of life and an open topic of conversation. Many of us did not grow up that way. Some of us never heard our parents openly talk about sexuality until we got "The Talk." Some of us were raised in a family that ignored or suppressed the topic of sexuality altogether. Others of us have memories of actively being shamed around the topic or being victims of sexual abuse. Whatever your experience, taking the time to think about your own history can be helpful. There are things that you may want to repeat and things that you may want to change in your own family.

In general, the purpose of this chapter is to help you identify the ways in which your past experiences and current attitudes about sexuality might impact your parenting. More specifically, we work toward three goals in this chapter: (a) to help you consider how you were raised and the values and attitudes you have today about sexuality, (b) to identify the values you want to teach your child, and (c) to help you identify areas of discomfort around sexuality so that you can work on them or get help if you need it. Working toward these three goals will help you to parent intentionally with an awareness of what, why, and how you are teaching your child. By taking time to think through your past and your beliefs, you can more easily make conscious decisions when you respond to your child. If you grew up in a family that was open about sexuality, this process may be easier for you than for others. But stick with us. We find that even the most educated and aware parents benefit from revisiting their ideas about sexuality.

LEARNING ABOUT SEXUALITY: A HISTORICAL PERSPECTIVE

Many parents feel guilty when their parenting behavior isn't what they consider to be ideal. When learning about sexuality, specifically, some parents can feel guilty that they haven't taught the right things or haven't responded perfectly to certain situations. But the aim isn't perfection. As you read, we urge you to be kind to yourself. If you are reading this book, it is because you have your child's best interest at heart. Like generations before us, parents today lack healthy models for how to talk openly about sexuality. Learning about the history of sexual attitudes in your community can help put individual families' behaviors about sex and sexuality into context.

Consider a popular book written by John Harvey Kellogg, first published in 1882, entitled *Plain Facts for Old and Young*. Its purpose was to educate society on the prevalence of sexual misconduct and to offer remedies for fixing them. In one section, Kellogg gave cures for childhood "self-abuse" (his term for masturbation), which included keeping the child occupied at all times; ensuring that the child is never left alone, including overnight; bandaging the genitals or covering them with a cage; tying the hands together; and performing a circumcision without the administration of anesthetic (Kellogg, 1882). Our purpose in mentioning Kellogg here is not to vilify him but to illustrate how much we have had to unlearn as a culture. We now know that masturbation is quite normal for people of every age, including young children. Although attitudes and knowledge about sexuality have changed since the 1880s, the ideas that Kellogg promoted remain part of our cultural history.

By the 1940s, along with the famous Kinsey studies on human sexuality (e.g., Kinsey et al., 1948), ideas about sexual health were changing. In his widely read books on baby and child care, for instance, Benjamin Spock recognized the normality of sexual behavior starting in infancy and contended—just as we do—that kids are learning about sexuality throughout the entirety of their childhoods. His recommendation was that talks about sexuality "come up from time to time" rather than in one big lecture (Spock, 2012, p. 723; see also Spock, 1946). Still, during the 1940s and 1950s, attitudes toward sexual health remained mostly focused on moral purity with goals, such as eliminating masturbation and premarital sexual behavior.

It wasn't until the 1960s and 1970s that changing attitudes toward sexuality in general began to have a greater positive effect on how we teach children about sexual health. In the 1980s, the AIDS epidemic further spurred a new effort to teach youth about sexuality (Elia, 2009). Over time, we also began to see the emergence of more evidence-based research into how to teach about sexual health most effectively. There is now clear evidence that parents can have a meaningful, positive impact on their child's sexual health when they have frequent, ongoing conversations with their child about sexuality (Martino et al., 2008). Moreover, sexual health educators agree that sexuality education begins in infancy whether we provide it intentionally or not (Breuner et al., 2016).

In recent decades, many books have become available to help parents teach their children about sexuality. These books are often full of accurate information based on current knowledge about sexuality and child development. Still, attitudes passed from generation to generation take time to change. More than a century and a half after Kellogg's ideas were being read, our effort to understand childhood sexuality and intentionally teach our children about it is still a work in progress. Our hope is that this book will be one more step toward a culture in which teaching about healthy sexuality from the beginning of a child's life is a consistent part of our culture.

A NOTE FOR DADS

As we have talked with parents, we have noticed that there is often a gender difference when it comes to teaching children about healthy sexuality. Dads have expressed that they *want* to tackle the tough topics with their child, but they feel they are working against social norms. They might feel more judged and uncomfortable for a plethora of different reasons, ranging from gender differences in general parenting duties to fears of being viewed as predatory or inappropriate. Whether your feelings of awkwardness are the result of personal history or cultural norms, they are worth investigating. If you are a dad and feel uncomfortable addressing sexuality topics with your child, take some time to consider why you feel the way you do.

As a result of gender disparities in parenting, dads who are coparenting with a woman often leave these topics for moms to address. In other families, dads take responsibility for talking with sons, while moms talk with daughters. Regardless of your coparenting status, there are extremely good reasons why it's important to buck the system and talk to your child yourself regardless of your child's gender. You have a unique perspective. You have your own feelings and attitudes around sexuality to share with your child. You are modeling behavior that your child will internalize. How are men and husbands and dads supposed to behave in relationships? How are they expected to communicate about sexuality? What are their attitudes toward affection, body image, emotions, or health? Your child is learning these things from you.

Moreover, you want your child to know that you have their back no matter what they're going through. When you are open about the hard topics, kids will learn that you are a parent who is approachable and who can talk with them about difficult or awkward situations. So, know that you're not alone. Talk with other dads if you can, and start now while your child is developing the foundations of their sexual health.

EXERCISES: EXPLORING YOUR HISTORY, FEELINGS, AND VALUES

How you say things can be just as important as what you say (or don't say!). Almost every parent has areas of sexuality with which they feel squeamish, and therefore, anxious. Because children detect and mirror spoken and unspoken anxieties, it is better to process your feelings ahead of time as much as possible to reduce, or at least accept, discomfort.

The exercises in this section are intended to help you consider your feelings about sexuality and discover areas you may benefit from thinking about more deeply. You might choose to do these now or you might choose to come back to them after you've finished reading the rest of Part I in this book. If you find yourself unsure of some of the language or content in these exercises, coming back to them before diving into Part II might be best for you. One approach is to read through all of the exercises first. Some will resonate with you, whereas others will not. Work through as many as you can. Completing at least one of them will have benefits for you and your child. After completing the exercises you choose, we guide you through options for what you can do next.

Exercise 1

The purpose of this exercise is to get the ball rolling, to help you to start thinking about your own sexuality and how you do or don't want to pass down your feelings and values to your child. Write your answers to the following questions as best you can. You can write your answers here, in a journal, on a computer, or any other place that feels good to you.

We recommend setting a 5-minute timer for each of these topics. Once the time is up, move on. If you haven't finished answering a question, you can come back to it later.

- Growing up, what verbal and nonverbal messages about sexuality did you receive from your parents, other family, school or friends, your community, and the media? (If you are having trouble thinking of topics, revisit the sexuality perspectives and models from Chapter 1.)

  _____

  _____

  _____

  _____

(continues)

(*continued*)

- Do you want to raise your children in the same way you were raised with regard to learning about sexuality? What things would you like to do the same? What things would you like to do differently?

  _____

  _____

  _____

  _____

- How do you feel about your own sexuality and sexual history? What parts of your sexuality do you feel good about? Are there parts of your sexuality or sexual history you wish you could change? Have you internalized any messages about sexuality that you would like to rewrite?

  _____

  _____

  _____

  _____

- Do you want to pass on to your child any parts of your own sexuality, current or historical? Are there parts of your own sexuality, current or historical, that you do not want your child to experience?

  _____

  _____

  _____

  _____

Now that you have finished answering these questions, take a minute and check in with your body. Have you been breathing deep, slow breaths? Has your breathing become shallow, or has it stopped? Do you feel relaxed? Do you have any tension in your body? If so, where are you feeling that tension? It is normal to have a range of feelings around these topics. You don't need to change those feelings, but it can be helpful to notice them and allow yourself the time to just sit with them for a few moments.

Before you move on, go back to your answers and highlight anything you'd like to work on more. Is there something you'd like to talk about with a friend, coparent, or therapist? Is there anything you'd like to pay special attention to as you read through this book?

Exercise 2

This exercise is intended to help you further recognize areas in which you could use a little more help getting comfortable or alleviating anxiety. Read each prompt and finish the sentence in your mind or by writing it down. Then check in with your body and notice your response. For some prompts, you might get a *zing* of adrenaline; for others, you might feel completely calm. If a prompt produces noticeable discomfort, put a check mark inside the box beside it.

☐ When I imagine my child saying the word *penis* to their teacher, I feel . . .

_____

_____

_____

_____

☐ When it comes to sex, I was taught that women are . . .

_____

_____

_____

_____

(continues)

(continued)

☐ With regard to gender roles, I was taught that men should . . .

_____
_____
_____
_____

☐ I feel most connected to a partner when . . .

_____
_____
_____
_____

☐ When I think about my child's sexuality, I am afraid that . . .

_____
_____
_____
_____

☐ When I imagine my child having the same body image I have of myself, I feel . . .

_____
_____
_____
_____

☐ I am worried that my child will . . .

_____
_____
_____
_____

☐ When I think of my child as a toddler masturbating, I feel . . .

_____
_____
_____
_____

☐ When I think of my child as a teenager masturbating, I feel . . .

_____
_____
_____
_____

☐ I am excited that my child will know _____ about sexuality.

_____
_____
_____
_____

☐ When I imagine my child doesn't want to hug their grandparent, I feel . . .

_____
_____
_____
_____

☐ If my child came out to me as gay, I would . . .

_____
_____
_____
_____

☐ When I think of my child as a teenager and becoming sexually active, I feel . . .

_____
_____
_____
_____

☐ When I think about sexual pleasure, I feel . . .

_____
_____
_____
_____

(*continues*)

(continued)

☐ My greatest hope for my child's sexuality is . . .

_____

_____

_____

_____

Now, say the following words out loud and consider how you feel when you say them. If a prompt produces noticeable discomfort, place a check mark inside the box beside it. (You will learn about these and more anatomical terms in Chapter 3.)

☐ Anus   ☐ Scrotum

☐ Clitoris   ☐ Vagina

☐ Penis   ☐ Vulva

When you have finished reviewing the preceding list, look back through the items that you selected with a check mark. Consider whether any of them deserve further investigation on your part so you may gain more clarity and comfort around them. If you do identify any topics for further inquiry, we have suggestions for you at the end of this chapter.

Exercise 3

Teaching young children about healthy sexuality will help them now and in the future. The purpose of this exercise is to help you focus on what you want for your child in the long run. In this exercise, we invite you to imagine your child is now a young adult, perhaps in their late 20s or 30s. When you think of the kind of person you hope your child will become *in general*, words may come to mind, such as *compassionate, courageous, flexible, fulfilled, generous, grounded, happy, resilient, successful,* or *thoughtful*. Healthy sexuality is a big part of being a healthy adult.

The following is a list of several aspects of sexuality. Read each item, one by one, and imagine your currently young child when they are years older, as a young adult, with regard to each topic. Write down the completed sentence here, on paper, or on a device of your choice.

• With regard to affection and physical comfort, I hope that my child . . .

_____

_____

_____

_____

• With regard to body image (i.e., awareness, comfort with, and appreciation of one's own body), I hope that my child . . .

_____

_____

_____

_____

• With regard to boundaries and consent (i.e., physical and emotional), I hope that my child . . .

_____

_____

_____

_____

• With regard to communication (i.e., the ability to discuss anatomy, bodily functions, feelings, and needs as well as understanding nonverbal communication), I hope that my child . . .

_____

_____

_____

_____

(continues)

(continued)

- With regard to compassion and empathy, I hope that my child . . .

  _____
  _____
  _____
  _____

- With regard to emotional intimacy (i.e., vulnerability, trust, and attachment), I hope that my child . . .

  _____
  _____
  _____
  _____

- With regard to expectations of a partner (i.e., what to expect from a dating relationship, committed relationship, or marriage/partnership), I hope that my child . . .

  _____
  _____
  _____
  _____

- With regard to gender roles and gender expression, I hope that my child . . .

  _____
  _____
  _____
  _____

- With regard to my expectations of when sexual behavior is appropriate (When are physical sexual interactions appropriate? Any time as long as it's responsible? Only in a committed relationship? Only after marriage?), I hope that my child . . .

  _____
  _____
  _____
  _____

- With regard to reproductive health (i.e., taking care of one's body medically, including awareness of sexually transmitted infection and contraception), I hope that my child . . .

  _____

  _____

  _____

  _____

- With regard to self-esteem and self-respect, I hope that my child . . .

  _____

  _____

  _____

  _____

- With regard to sexual orientation, I hope that my child . . .

  _____

  _____

  _____

  _____

- With regard to sexual pleasure (e.g., giving and receiving, enjoyment of one's own body, enjoyment of another's body), I hope that my child . . .

  _____

  _____

  _____

  _____

- With regard to spirituality (e.g., faith, cultural morality, social justice, rights), I hope that my child . . .

  _____

  _____

  _____

  _____

Now that you have completed the sentences, here are some questions to consider. Did any topics cause you to feel particularly confident or uncomfortable? Are there any topics in particular that you would like to focus on as you read through the rest of the book? Are there topics you know you would like to learn about more? Make note of your answers. You can come back to them once you've finished reading the book and see if your new knowledge has changed any of your perspectives.

Whether by example or through explicit verbal communication, we teach our children, starting at a very young age, about everything on this list. This book aims to help you to communicate about all of these topics with your child. But remember: This is just the beginning. The bigger idea is to open up lines of communication so that your child feels comfortable talking with you about these topics for years to come.

After You Have Completed Your Exercises

Are there topics or words in these three exercises that you were excited about? What about some that caused you to feel nervous or uneasy? Maybe there were topics or words that were distressing. All of these responses are normal. Sexuality can be a charged topic, and we all have different histories with our family, school, and society that shape how we feel about it.

Even sexual health educators, including us, your authors, are not immune to getting nervous about sexual topics. It took Laura ages to say the word *anus* to her child without feeling weird about it. She committed to using the term when it was appropriate, and over time, the term became comfortable for her. The same can happen for you too. You *can* become more comfortable with sexual topics.

Here are other suggestions for how to process those uncomfortable feelings and past experiences:

- **Go back and see if any of the topics *were* comfortable and easy for you.** Even if you can find just one, you can build on that. If there are many comfortable topics, that's great.
- **Talk with your coparent, if you have one.** Being on the same page with your coparent—and even agreeing on who will talk with your child about what topics—is powerful and ultimately helpful for your coparenting journey.
- **Consider talking with a trusted friend or group of friends about your answers.** We find that hearing about others' experiences and telling about your own can help to understand, or process, your feelings. You may also realize that you're not alone in feeling uncomfortable or upset. Talking with others also helps a person get used to discussing these topics out loud and solidify what they think about them.
- **Practice.** If you feel uncomfortable saying a particular word, practice saying the word out loud. Try saying the word 100 times out loud and then see if it feels any different to you.
- **Educate yourself on topics about which you feel less confident.** This book includes information on what you'll need to know when you talk to young children. You can also find videos, podcasts, websites, and other resources that address these topics, many of which are listed in the Resources sections found in most chapters of this book.
- **Spend more time writing about uncomfortable topics in a journal (or wherever feels best to you).** Consider *why* these topics make you feel the way they do.
- **See a therapist.** Therapists are trained to help people process topics like these and provide accurate information. They are a wonderful resource. Therapy may be particularly helpful for those who know they have experienced sexual trauma in the past or are finding themselves "flooded" or overwhelmed with their feelings during these exercises.

- Remember that when you start teaching your child about sexuality at the earliest ages (before about age 5 years), *they* will not be embarrassed or uncomfortable. That means it's the perfect time for you to ease into a topic and get used to it.

SUMMARY

- It is normal to feel nervous about discussing sexuality with your child. The more informed you are and the more you practice doing it, the more comfortable you will become. We are hopeful that this book will also help you to feel more confident when talking with your child.
- Sometimes a parent doesn't know what will trigger strong feelings until they are faced with a particular situation.
- Taking time to think through your history and beliefs will help you to respond in a more intentional way and reduce your reactivity.
- The three exercises we have provided are intended to help you consider your own history, more clearly identify the values you have and want to pass on, and help you find topics for which you may want to spend a bit more time processing.
- We have several recommendations once you have identified areas of sexuality for which you need more time or help to process. These include building on your strengths and what you are already comfortable with, talking with a coparent and trusted friends, practicing, educating yourself on specific topics, writing in a journal, seeing a therapist, and remembering that you have time to get more comfortable.

RESOURCES FOR PARENTS

Online

- American Psychological Association therapist locator: https:// locator.apa.org

- Brené Brown's TED talk on shame: https://www.ted.com/talks/brene_brown_listening_to_shame?language=en
- Society for Sex Therapy & Research therapist locator: https://sstarnet.org/find-a-therapist/

Books

- *Come as You Are: The Surprising New Science That Will Transform Your Sex Life* by Emily Nagoski (Simon & Schuster Paperbacks)
- *The Courage to Heal: A Guide for Women Survivors of Child Sexual Abuse* (4th ed.) by Ellen Bass and Laura Davis (Collins Living)
- *The Mindful Self-Compassion Workbook: A Proven Way to Accept Yourself, Build Inner Strength, and Thrive* by Kristin Neff and Christopher Germer (Guilford Press)

Chapter 3
Reproductive Anatomy and Physiology

As we discussed in Chapter 1, sexuality is about so much more than body parts. That said, the *anatomy* (body parts) and *physiology* (how the body parts work) of reproduction are an important part of what we will teach our kids about sexuality. Reproductive anatomy and physiology also include some of the topics that make parents most uncomfortable when they think of teaching their child about sexuality. At the same time, genitals are particularly fascinating to young (and older) children. There's a reason the game "You Show Me Yours and I'll Show You Mine" is so well known. Many times over, we have heard stories of children wanting to see the genitals of other children, especially when those genitals are different from their own. Children also want to know how things work. Why do penises get hard? How does the baby get into the belly in the first place? Why don't mommy's breasts make milk anymore? While you may not feel ready to tackle these types of situations and questions, getting familiar with accurate terminology now will help you be more comfortable when teaching your child.

Every person, including young children, lives inside a body that has all kinds of functions that can be confusing and even surprising and scary when they aren't understood. For each person to have a clear understanding of the way that their own body works and shapes the way they experience life is fundamental to their being able to have autonomy and control over themselves. This may be true for human sexuality more than any other human experience.

This chapter outlines reproductive anatomy and physiology about all bodies. People need to know about their own body and the bodies that other people have (Daly & O'Sullivan, 2020). In Part II of this book, we are specific about which terms you can teach your child and when. For now, take the time to familiarize yourself with sexual anatomy and language here. Regardless of the composition of your family, it is important that children learn about the reproductive anatomy of all people because this is the honest and accurate description of reproduction.

BIOLOGICAL SEX AND THE BINARY

Biological sex refers to the physical body and is defined using the terms *female*, *intersex*, or *male*.

The words "female" and "male" are shorthand words that indicate a specific collection and organization of anatomical features. However, these words often do not always describe the actuality of someone's reproductive anatomy or their gender identity.

The characteristic that is typically used to assign a baby's sex at birth is the *external genitalia* (the presence of a vulva or penis and scrotum). Importantly, however, a person's biological sex is actually not based on just one element or characteristic, and external genitalia are not always as clearly binary as popular culture suggests they are. Instead, each person's biological sex is based on the interplay of several characteristics, including

- external genitalia,
- internal reproductive anatomy,
- chromosomes,

- hormones, and
- secondary sexual characteristics, such as body hair or voice (Parent & Rayne, 2020).[1]

While most people find that their characteristics in these five categories all fall fairly neatly into one of two common patterns (female or male), many do not. When a person's physical sexual characteristics fall into patterns outside of the standard pattern of female or male characteristics, their biological sex is called *intersex*. Almost 2% of the population is intersex, depending on how the word *intersex* is defined. To put this number into context, approximately the same percentage of people are intersex as the percentage of people who have green eyes.

The development of a human fetus is astonishingly complicated, and there are numerous ways that intersex development happens. Intersex individuals often have either a variation in their genes or in the sex hormones present during development. For instance, an individual may have a more typical XX (female) or XY (male) genotype, but the fetus is exposed to unusual levels of hormones that disrupt the maturity of their reproductive anatomy. Alternatively, an individual may have an anomalous genotype, such as XYY or XXX. Signs that an infant may be intersex include ambiguous external genitalia, such as a very small penis, undescended testes, or an enlarged clitoris. An older child may discover they are intersex when they experience delayed, absent, or atypical puberty patterns, whereas some adults become aware of being intersex when they encounter problems with fertility.

Understanding the development of biological sex is useful as you teach your child about reproductive anatomy and physiology.

---

[1] All biological information presented in this chapter comes from Parent and Rayne (2020).

Kids are fascinated by how the body works, and even young children are capable of understanding that there is more to biological sex than external genitalia. When we teach children about the complexities of human biology, we invite them to appreciate the vast and beautiful biological variations within each of us. Furthermore, this approach is part of teaching your child to be inclusive of those whose sexual characteristics do not fall into a common pattern. Just as we work to raise people who don't discriminate based on nationality, sexual orientation, or disability, we can raise people who are accepting of all bodies.

REPRODUCTIVE ANATOMY

Understanding the names and functions of their body parts, including the sexual and reproductive parts, offers children ownership and appreciation of their body, autonomy in decision making, protection against sexual abuse, and a scaffolding that supports their ability to understand sexual consent in critical ways. The terms and definitions listed here are ones that young children need to know. We have provided you with both caregiver definitions (to describe the nuances to you) as well as language that you can use with your young child.

While all of this information is important for children to learn over time, it is best learned spread out over many conversations rather than all at once. Keep in mind that while we want to offer our child accurate information, the bigger picture is to establish an ongoing dialogue. You might not get it right every time, and that's okay. When we provide information using many small conversations over time, we have the opportunity for do-overs. (More specific information about how to teach your child about anatomy and physiology is provided in Part II.)

External Female Genitalia

Like the rest of the body, external female genitalia can vary dramatically in appearance. The size and shape of the inner labia, in particular,

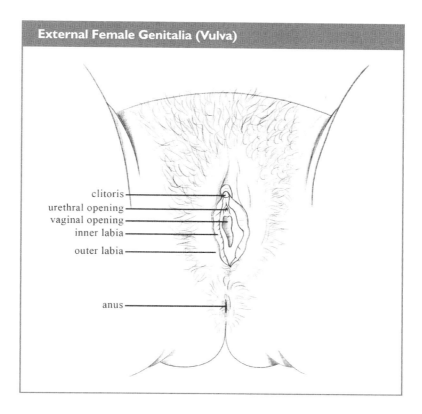

External Female Genitalia (Vulva)

clitoris
urethral opening
vaginal opening
inner labia
outer labia
anus

can be quite different from person to person. Later on, when your child is older, you will want to discuss these anatomical differences with them (see the figure *External Female Genitalia [Vulva]*). For now, just be aware that a wide range of variation is normal.

ANUS

The *anus* is the orifice of the body where feces exit the *rectum*, or bowels. The anus has social stigma associated with it. However, it is a normal part of everyone's body, and knowing how it works and what it does is important to many young children. Some people, but not all, find stimulation of the anus to be pleasurable. This includes young children. Pleasure from anal stimulation is a natural function of the nerve endings inside and around the anus and is not related to the person's sexual orientation or gender.

 What you can say:

"The anus is where poop comes out. It is the same for all people."

BREASTS

Although breasts are not part of reproductive anatomy, they are associated with birth and sexual response, and they also carry a lot of cultural meaning. Breasts are associated with breastfeeding, mothering, and sexual desire. In the United States, breasts are considered private, like genitals, and are a part of anatomy that is usually covered while in public. Breasts consist of mammary glands and fat, and they produce milk after the birth of an infant. Both male and female individuals have mammary tissue. Nipples are highly innervated, and touching them can be pleasurable regardless of one's biological sex.

 What you can say:

"Breasts grow during puberty for many people. For people with a uterus, they stay past puberty and are a permanent part of their body. Often when a baby is born, breasts produce milk to feed the baby. The nipples on breasts and chests can be very sensitive and feel good or soothing to touch."

CLITORIS

The *clitoris* is a sex organ with the sole purpose of experiencing pleasure. Although the part of the clitoris that we see externally is quite small, the majority of the organ is found inside the body. At the beginning of fetal development, all fetuses have the same types of tissue. Depending on the chromosomes and hormones present, the fetus will usually develop into either a male or female. In that case, the phallus tissue either becomes a clitoris, which is mostly internal, or a penis, which is mostly external. Both the clitoris and the penis have a *glans*, or head, and tissue that covers the head. The tissue covering the head is called the *foreskin* of the penis or *hood* of the clitoris. The pea-sized glans of the clitoris has a high concentration of nerve endings and is very sensitive. Stimulation of clitoris (either internally via the vagina or externally via the glans) produces orgasm in many females.

 What you can say:

"The clitoris is a small bump toward the top of the vulva. It's very sensitive. For some people, it feels good to touch the clitoris, and for others, it doesn't. Either way is fine."

LABIA

The *labia* are sensitive folds of skin that surround and protect the clitoris, urethral opening, and vaginal opening. There are two sets of labia: the external (or outer), which are on the outside, and the internal (or inner), which are on the inside. Either one of these can be larger than the other.

 What you can say:

"The folds of skin that protect your vagina, clitoris, and opening to the urethra are called your labia."

URETHRAL OPENING

About midway down the vulva is a tiny opening to the urethra. The *urethral opening* is where urine exits the body. It is important to be aware of the difference between the urethral opening and the vaginal opening.

 What you can say:

"There's a tiny hole about in the middle of the vulva where pee comes out. That's the opening to the urethra."

55

VULVA

The *vulva* comprises all the external genitalia of a female person, including the labia, clitoris, urethral opening, and vaginal opening. The word *vulva* is commonly used to identify all of these visible parts, but the labia are what we can see the most clearly. The terms *vulva* and *vagina* are often confused. The vagina is entirely internal (and is described in detail later in the Internal Female Reproductive Organs section of this chapter). Externally, we can see the vaginal opening, but we cannot see the vagina itself. When we refer to the female genitals that a child can see, we can call them the vulva. Using the term *vagina* when referring to what we can see on the outside is incorrect. (That said, we applaud parents who use the term in an effort to avoid using slang terms for genitals!)

 What you can say:

"The vulva is the part of the body between a female person's legs. For some people, it feels good to touch the different parts of the vulva, and for others, it doesn't. Either way is fine. Your vulva is only for you to touch. Sometimes I may need to touch it, but only if you need help for some medical reason. A doctor might need to help you with your genitals as well, but they should only do that if a trusted adult is with you."

Internal Female Reproductive Organs

In this section, as with the rest of this chapter, we provide you with accurate anatomical terms. The terms for internal female reproductive organs will be relevant when you discuss topics like differences among female, intersex, and male bodies, or how babies are made. Rather than telling your child that the baby grows in a "belly," you can use the term *uterus*, for example. This may seem like too much information for a toddler or even a kindergartner, and indeed, the terms will need repeating time after time (see the figure *Internal Female Reproductive Organs*).

56

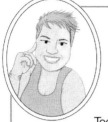

Allegra
BROOKLYN PARK, MINNESOTA

Mother to two children
Age when first child was born: 29

Today, the girls got to meet my cousin Natalie's new baby, Kate! She is the most adorable thing. Both girls were entranced with baby Kate. We did have one pretty wild moment, though.

Not being able to breastfeed either of the girls when they were babies didn't bother me too much. It was hard sometimes, since my coworkers with babies were able to breastfeed so easily. But since I couldn't breastfeed, and my close friends aren't parents yet, my girls haven't really seen breastfeeding happen, unless it has been with a cover over the baby. I know they have heard people talk about breastfeeding, but I guess I didn't realize how little they knew. My cousin has been living in Europe since before baby Kate was born, and where she lives, breastfeeding in public is super common. At the restaurant we were at, Kate started crying, and Natalie undid her nursing top and began feeding her without a cover. The girls had extremely different reactions to what was happening. The 3-year-old was extremely concerned at first and thought the baby was eating Natalie! I am serious—she literally said, "Stop it baby! Stop eating Auntie Nat! You are a zombie!" This was met with a mix of laughter from some restaurant guests and extremely rude glares from others. I mean, come on! She's 3! What do you expect?!

My older girl, on the other hand, watched very curiously and quietly until Kate was done nursing and Natalie was buttoning back up her shirt. She walked over to Natalie and said, "So, you're like a soda machine kind of. Does anything else come out besides milk?"

Thank God Nat has a sense of humor! I really have to do a little more educating with these gals around anatomy (and apparently also zombies).

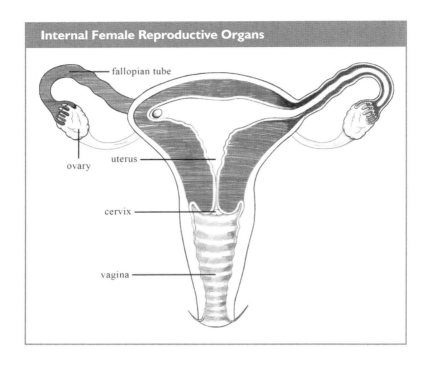

Internal Female Reproductive Organs

fallopian tube

ovary

uterus

cervix

vagina

There are several reasons we want to use these terms starting early in childhood. First, we want to make it clear that terms related to genitals and reproduction are viewed as normal and not embarrassing. Second, when we start teaching these terms early, it makes our job easier down the road. For instance, as children get older, they will want more details about how things like conception work. A 6-year-old might ask a more complex question, such as, "Can a person not have a baby if they don't want one?" When children have already heard terms, such as *uterus* and *vagina*, it's easier and clearer to add information to what they already know. And third, knowing correct terminology avoids confusion about how the body works.

Karen has seen frequent confusion among children, teenagers, and even young adults about things like whether a growing fetus eats actual food from the stomach of the pregnant person or whether someone can get pregnant from oral sex. Identifying the differences between the digestive and reproductive systems early on helps to prevent this kind of confusion.

CERVIX

The *cervix* is the lower part of the uterus and functions as a gateway to and from the uterus and vagina. It produces cervical fluid, which is discharged throughout the month when a female person is not menstruating.

 What you can say:

"This is the part of the uterus that opens into the vagina for a baby to be born."

FALLOPIAN TUBES

Fallopian tubes connect the ovaries to the uterus. However, they are not fully connected to the ovaries. Instead, little hairlike projections called *cilia* scoop up eggs that are released from the ovaries and bring them into the fallopian tubes. The fallopian tubes are where conception occurs if fertilization of an egg happens inside the body.

 What you can say:

"Fallopian tubes are how an egg gets from the ovary to the uterus."

OVARIES

The *ovaries* produce hormones, such as estrogen and progesterone, and are the place where eggs mature and are released.

What you can say:

"Ovaries are where eggs are made. (They aren't like chicken eggs, though!) Eggs are necessary for a pregnancy to happen. Most people who have ovaries have two of them, one on each side of their body."

URETHRA

The *urethra* is the tube that runs from the bladder to the urethral opening. It most often carries urine out from the bladder. The urethra is separate from the vagina. (The urethra is not pictured in the drawing. It is in front of the vagina.)

 What you can say:

"The urethra is the tube where pee can come down from the bladder and out of the body."

UTERUS

The *uterus* is where a fetus gestates. The uterus is typically the size of a person's fist, and over the 40 weeks of pregnancy, it grows into the largest muscle in the pregnant person's body. During childbirth, the uterus is the muscle that contracts, opening the cervix, and eventually pushing the baby out through the vagina.

 What you can say:

"The uterus is where a fetus grows into a baby. It is located right in the middle of the body above the bladder."

VAGINA

The *vagina* is a muscular tube between the vulva and the cervix. In the context of pregnancy, it is often referred to as the *birth canal*, but countless other slang terms are also used when referring to the vagina. As mentioned earlier, however, the vagina should not be confused with the vulva. The vagina is where menstrual fluid comes out of the body during menstruation. Many (although definitely not all) people with vaginas enjoy having them penetrated during sexual activity.

What you can say:

"The vagina is a stretchy tube that connects the uterus to the vulva so the baby can come all the way out of the pregnant person's body. It is also where menstrual fluid comes out during a period."

Allegra
BROOKLYN PARK, MINNESOTA

Mother to two children
Age when first child was born: 29

Despite being so young, Violet has had a lot of questions about reproductive anatomy lately. So, while I had the girls with me at work today, I gave them an anatomy worksheet to color. The two went out into our waiting room with the water dispenser and the rocking moose (not a horse, a moose, from IKEA), and I heard them giggling and singing, but I couldn't make out the words. I was finally ready to leave, got the girls buckled into car seats, and hit the road. Except by hitting the road, I mean hitting gridlock traffic at rush hour. I always prefer fresh air, so we had the windows rolled down, and suddenly, as if rehearsed, an EXTREMELY loud song came from the back seat, which sounded like, "Unerus, unerus, we've got a unerus! Unerus, unerus, looks like a naked moose. Unerus, unerus, unerus, unerus, it's pink and it looks like jelly." I realized they meant "uterus!" I looked back, trying not to die laughing, and I see that, out of nowhere, Violet has pulled out a uterus picture that she has drawn a smiling face on and taped to a pencil and is waving it around like a rhythmic gymnast, while Stella has rolled down her window and is shrieking (to the car stopped DIRECTLY next to us), "We have three unerusis in our car! How many are in your car?!"

(continues)

(*continued*)

> Try as I might, we were not able to move immediately, nor did the earth swallow us whole, nor were my daughters able to get the entire highway to do a group singalong of "The Unerus Song," try as they might.
>
> We did finally make it home, and I know that the unerus song will be a family favorite for years to come.

External Male Genitalia

This section provides you with accurate terms for external male genitals. Just like the terms used for female anatomy, there are many slang terms used for male genitalia. It's not necessary to strictly outlaw such terms in your home (as long as they are respectful), but do your best to use accurate terms equally as often (see the figure *External Male Genitalia*).

Anus

See the definition in the earlier section on external female genitalia.

Foreskin

Covering the glans of the penis is the *foreskin*. Some penises are surgically circumcised, usually very near birth, removing the foreskin. Many people feel very strongly about circumcision—either for or against it—for religious, medical, or social reasons. There is no immediate medical need for a normally formed penis to be circumcised. Although there are some minor medical benefits to circumcision, such as a slightly lower rate of sexually transmitted infections for people with a circumcised penis, there are also minor risks to the procedure.

 What you can say:

"This is skin that covers the tip of a penis. Some penises have had that skin removed."

External Male Genitalia

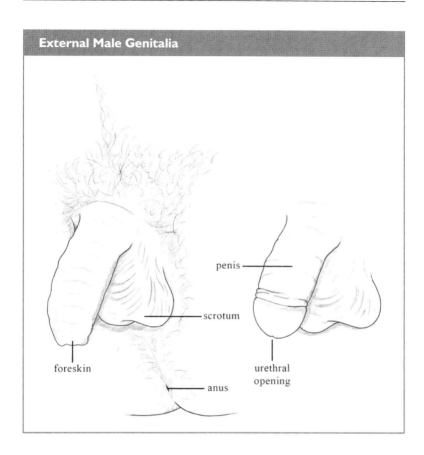

penis

scrotum

foreskin

urethral opening

anus

URETHRAL OPENING

At the end of the penis is an opening to the urethra. This *urethral opening* is where either semen or urine exit the body.

 What you can say:

> "At the end of the penis, there is an opening to the urethra. This is where pee comes out. It's also how sperm get out of the body."

63

PENIS

The *penis* is part of the external male genitalia. It extends from the body just above where the legs meet. As we discussed earlier, all fetuses begin with the same types of genital tissue during fetal development. The fetus then usually develops into either a male or female person, depending on the chromosomes and hormones present. The phallus tissue either becomes a *clitoris*, which is mostly internal, or a penis, which is mostly external. Both the clitoris and the penis have a *glans*, or head, and tissue that covers the head. The tissue covering the head is called the foreskin of the penis or *hood* of the clitoris. Inside the penis are two kinds of tissue called the *corpus cavernosum* and the *corpus spongiosum* that will fill with blood and harden. This is what makes the penis erect. Stimulation of the penis produces orgasm in many males.

 What you can say:

"The penis is a body part that comes out just above where the legs meet. For some people, it feels good to touch the penis, and for others, it doesn't. Either way is fine. Sometimes when penises are touched, they get larger and harder. Your penis is only for you to touch. Sometimes I may need to touch it, but only if you need help for some medical reason. A doctor might need to help you with your genitals as well, but they should only do that if a trusted adult is with you."

SCROTUM

Many people refer to the sacs under the penis as "testicles." While there are testicles inside, what we actually see is the *scrotum*. Naming the inside and outside anatomy differently is important for young children as they learn to understand their bodies and in the event that they need help with some element of their genitals. (As with the confusion over the terms *vulva* and *vagina*, misunderstanding anatomical terms is common. If you have been using the term *testicles* instead of *scrotum*, we are pleased that you are making an effort to use anatomically correct terms in the first place!)

 What you can say:

> "The scrotum is skin that hangs down beneath the penis and holds the testicles."

Internal Male Reproductive Organs

Your last sex ed anatomy lesson is about internal male reproductive organs (see the figure). Both the internal female and male reproductive organs shown in this chapter have many more organs

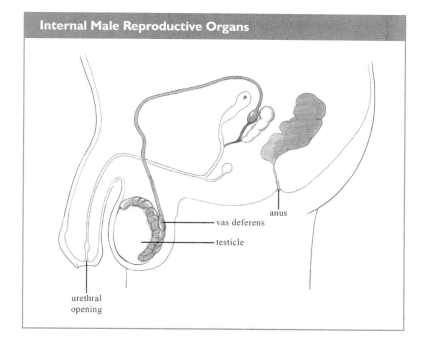

Internal Male Reproductive Organs

vas deferens

anus

testicle

urethral opening

than what we have labeled. If you're interested in learning more, we have provided a resource at the end of this chapter.

TESTICLES

Located inside the scrotum, the *testicles*, also called "testes," produce both sperm and hormones. Closely attached to the testes are the *epididymis*, which is where the sperm mature and wait until an ejaculation is imminent.

 What you can say:

"Testes are where sperm are made. Sperm are necessary for a pregnancy to happen. Most people who have testes have two of them, hanging below their penis inside the scrotum."

URETHRA

The *urethra* is the tube that runs from the bladder and meets with the vas deferens. It then goes through the penis and can carry either sperm or urine. Semen and urine cannot pass through the urethra at the same time.

 What you can say:

"The urethra is a tube that comes out from the bladder. It is also connected to a tube that goes to the testes. Either pee or sperm can come down through this tube in the middle of the penis to get out of the body, but not at the same time."

VAS DEFERENS

The *vas deferens* is the tube that carries semen from the testes to the urethra, through which it is ejaculated. The vas deferens is what is cut during a vasectomy.

What you can say:

"The vas deferens is the tube that takes sperm from the testes to the urethra, where they can come out of the body."

Will

EASTON, PENNSYLVANIA

Father to two children
Age when first child was born: 30

    I taught Ryan and Connor accurate names of body parts. They were among the few young children who knew the more encompassing term *vulva*, whereas other children learn *vagina*, and many learn baby words or nothing. Years ago, Ryan corrected his cousin, who had proudly announced that girls have vaginas and boys have penises. Both certain they were correct, they sought out grandma to resolve the dispute, who promptly referred them to me.

    Everyone in the family can always count on me for honest and complete answers to their questions. I'm glad of that because I know it's not the same for everyone. My friend Jonathan is an example. I guess he was concerned about his family and friends seeing his newborn's nudity because the album contains dozens of strategically placed Post-it notes concealing her genitals and buttocks. Infants are, of course, very small, and Post-it notes—even the mini ones—take up a lot of space on a newborn's body. So, we were able to see her face, hands, feet, and some of her arms and legs but mostly other people in the photos—all smiling and not as concerned about her nudity. Even at my house, he always turns over any books that might have the word "sex."

    All of this misinformation or hidden information just isn't good for anyone.

REPRODUCTIVE PHYSIOLOGY—THAT IS, HOW BABIES GET MADE

At birth, the ovaries contain all the eggs they will have for a lifetime. In fact, lots of the initial egg cells die before puberty. Beginning during puberty, one egg a month on average develops to maturity and is released into the body cavity. A fallopian tube then catches the egg and pushes it down toward the uterus.

A person with a uterus and fertile egg supply gets their period, or menstruates, about once a month. Throughout the month, a fresh blood supply lines the walls of the uterus in preparation for a pregnancy. If no pregnancy occurs, the body purges this uterine lining through the cervix and vagina.

Testes, on the other hand, begin to make sperm in a continuous process during puberty and lasting throughout life. Sperm exit the body in a liquid called *semen*, or *ejaculate*.

To make a baby, a sperm has to enter an egg, and the resulting fertilized egg needs a uterus in which to grow. There are several different ways that an egg and sperm can get together, implant in a uterus, and make a baby.

Insemination

During *insemination*, sperm from one person are inserted into the vagina, uterus, or fallopian tubes of another person. The most common method is intrauterine insemination, or IUI.

 What you can say:

"A doctor or a nurse can take sperm from one person and put them into another person's vagina, uterus, or fallopian tubes, where they will wait for an egg to be released."

Intercourse

Penile–vaginal intercourse is when a penis gets erect and is inserted into a vagina. When this happens, and the penis feels good and orgasms, it releases a fluid called ejaculate that carries sperm. Sperm can then travel through the cervix and uterus into the fallopian tubes, where they wait for an egg to be released from the ovary. Only one sperm is usually able to enter an egg. Once this happens, the fertilized egg, or *zygote*, is pushed back down the fallopian tube and eventually implants in the lining of the uterus, where it can start to grow into a baby.

 What you can say:

> "Sometimes an adult with a vagina and an adult with a penis come together so that the penis goes inside the vagina. The penis can then release sperm into the vagina. The sperm can then swim all the way up through the cervix and the uterus to the fallopian tubes, where they can meet with an egg. After the sperm and the egg meet, they go back down the fallopian tube to the uterus and can start to grow into a baby."

In Vitro Fertilization

Through a medical procedure called *in vitro fertilization*, a physician can remove eggs from an ovary. The eggs are mixed or injected with sperm in a laboratory to become fertilized. One or more fertilized eggs are then transferred to a uterus.

 What you can say:

> "A doctor can do a procedure on a person with ovaries to get eggs out of the ovary. Then the doctor mixes them with sperm and puts them into a person's uterus."

Surrogacy

Sometimes a person or persons wishing to have a baby are unable to carry a pregnancy themselves. This can be because they don't have a uterus or for other medical reasons. In this case, *surrogacy* can be used: A person with a uterus can be hired as, or volunteers to be, a surrogate to gestate the baby. The egg and sperm used in this process come from people other than the surrogate.

What you can say:

"This is when a person or persons want to have a baby, but they don't have a uterus or their uterus can't grow a baby. A doctor takes sperm and eggs, like with IVF, and puts them into the body of another person who does have a uterus that can grow a baby."

Maya
AMSTERDAM, THE NETHERLANDS

Mother to one child
Age when child was born: 41

Chloe has started asking more questions about where babies come from and how they are made. What do I say to a 3-year-old? Mom and Dad were always *very* honest with us about that. Mom actually told me more recently that when she was little, Grandma and Grandpa would tell her things like "I will tell you when you are bigger" or just plain lies about the stork and other stories. That made Mom so angry that she decided she would never do that to her children. That's why she told my sisters and me all the details about baby-making from such a young age! I remember being a little grossed out with the whole lovemaking part of the story. I think that part was maybe too much, too soon.

So now, it's interesting to be making my own decisions about what to tell Chloe. She has been asking these questions for about a year, and she's now starting to understand more. In general, I want to tell her the honest answers to her questions but with just the right amount of information for her little 3-year-old brain to process. At first, I just told her babies come from an egg and a seed and that they grow in their mommies' bellies. That satisfied her early on. She loved to play that she was a pregnant mommy and put dolls and stuffed animals under her shirt. (Sometimes she would even sleep the whole night with a snuggle stuffed under her pajamas!) Now, she's asking the next level of questions, like, "Can we go to the store and buy some of those seeds?" She really wants a baby sister because her friend just got one. I explained to her that these seeds come from daddies and that they can't be bought. Now, she wants to play being pregnant, and she says, "Mommy can you be the daddy and put the seed in my tummy so I can have a baby?" She is thinking it is something that you could just put in there like planting a seed in the garden with your hands. She also asked, "How do the babies come out of the belly?" I told her that they come out of your vagina—that there is a "pee-hole" and a "baby-hole." She seems satisfied with these answers. I'll add more new details to the story as she grows older and asks for them, but for now, I'm feeling good about my approach.

DO I *REALLY* NEED TO KNOW THIS STUFF?

All of this anatomical and physiological language can seem very technical. Why do parents need to know all this when their kid is running around in diapers? There are many situations in which sexual anatomy and physiology come up during early childhood (Allen et al., 2018). Foremost, if you have an inquisitive and verbal child, they will ask you direct questions. Even if your child isn't a chatterbox, early childhood is full of opportunities to teach them about bodies and how they work. Whether it's diaper changes, bath time, beach time, or when your child is exploring their genitals, you can take advantage of everyday teaching opportunities. But why? Kids who know about their body, such as proper anatomical names for genitalia and appropriate boundaries for them, feel a greater ownership over, and pride in, their own body; are better protected against child sexual abuse; know that they can talk to caregivers about their whole body in case they need help; and are less likely to experience shame associated with sexual topics. Another reason why we recommend telling young kids about sexual anatomy and physiology is because it sets a precedent: All people deserve to have accurate, fact-based knowledge about sexuality (Daly & O'Sullivan, 2020). By starting when your child is young, you set them up to expect open, honest information in years to come.

Despite all these reasons to teach children about sexual anatomy, it can be hard. As we discussed in Chapter 2, most of us have grown up in a culture with a great stigma around sexuality. For many of us, talking about these topics can be uncomfortable or triggering. Keep in mind that your child is not yet embarrassed by these terms and ideas. By talking openly about sexuality with your child, you are working toward ending a cycle of shame around the topic. Know that you're not alone. Talk with other parents about their experiences and how they want to raise their children, and get professional help if you're feeling overwhelmed by this material. And keep up the good work! The more you discuss these topics with your child and others, the more comfortable you will become.

Melissa
ASHEVILLE, NORTH CAROLINA

Mother to two children
Age when first child was born: 29

The other day in the bath, River hid his penis between his legs so we couldn't see it at all and was squirming around, saying, "Mommy, look at my vulva. I'm a girl! I don't have a penis anymore. I turned into a girl!" He was clearly delighting in that idea, and I'm always vaguely curious about his gender identity but generally take it in stride and just let him be himself.

But then, penis still hidden, he launched into a series of questions about girls and boys and penises and vulvas—what they're all for, why we don't all have both, etc. I answered as honestly and simply as I could, which seemed enough for him at the time.

While I thought the conversation went well, I also noticed that I really, REALLY didn't want to get into the details of penis-in-vagina sex yet. He loves the book *What Makes a Baby*,[2] which is beautifully inclusive and sufficient (for a toddler at least) about the actual baby-making aspects of sperm and egg. But when should I tell him about sexual intercourse? I was totally taken off guard! He eventually shifted to another topic, but I'm still uncertain about how to deal with this.

As far back as I remember, I always knew about sex. And that also meant that I played all kinds of sexual games with my friends at this age and was sexually abused by a much older boy (and later a man). I went along with it because I had the idea that sex is a natural, good part of life, and my mom said it was beautiful . . . but without clarifying the need for mutual consent or which activities were not appropriate for me to engage in at that age.

And now, I'm afraid if I tell my son too much about sex (like even the penis-in-vagina concept), that could give him ideas that he doesn't already have, which could lead to the kinds of inappropriate sexual behaviors I experienced, especially since most of his best friends are girls. I want to protect other little girls in ways I wasn't protected! But I also want my son to know what he needs to know and not hear it from other kids or random people. How do I find the right time line and balance to share information in an age-appropriate, safe way?

SUMMARY

- Reproductive anatomy and physiology are an important part of teaching about sexuality. Using correct terminology for genitals is beneficial for children and may help to keep them safer from sexual abuse.

---

[2] *What Makes a Baby* by Cory Silverberg (Triangle Square).

- While children are particularly curious about genitals and how the body works, parents are often uncomfortable with these topics. Familiarizing yourself with the terms and concepts in this chapter can be helpful.
- The biological sex of a person—female, male, or intersex—is based on the interplay of several characteristics and is not binary.
- Any of the terms or concepts in this chapter can be discussed with young children using developmentally appropriate language.
- When discussing reproduction, we can start with the basics: A baby is made when the egg from one person comes together with the sperm of another person and then grows in a uterus. When the time comes, it is helpful to explain that there are many ways we bring babies into a family, including insemination, intercourse, IVF, and surrogacy. (Although adoption is not technically a biological process, and therefore not part of this chapter, it is important to discuss adoption either in the context of conception or when discussing different kinds of families.)

RESOURCES FOR PARENTS

- *How Do I Talk With My Preschooler About Their Body?* Planned Parenthood: https://www.plannedparenthood.org/learn/parents/preschool/how-do-i-talk-my-preschooler-about-their-body
- *Human Sexuality: Diversity in Contemporary Society* (10th edition) by William Yarber and Barbara Sayad (McGraw Hill)

Chapter 4
Gender and Sexual Orientation

Our collective, cultural understanding of gender and sexual identity is evolving at breakneck speed. Even in the past 5 years, our understanding of sexual orientation and gender has shifted in interesting and dramatic ways. We do not expect this trend to slow down in the near future, although we assume that, at some point, the evolution of understanding our own identities will plateau. Until then, it is critical to understand that any written perspective on sexual identity is a product of the time and place where it was written and by whom. We are both cis,[1] White, women: one lesbian and one bisexual. We live in the United States and Europe. We understand that both identity and sexuality are deeply culturally bound. This is one perspective on sexual identity that has been supported by academic psychological research on a global level. We hope it provides context and utility for you in your evolving understanding of gender and sexual orientation.

The fast pace of change in ideas around gender in particular can be a challenge for parents. Growing up, most of us were taught some version of: "Boys and men have a penis and are masculine; girls and

---

[1]The term *cis-* refers to people whose gender identity and gender expression correspond to their biological sex.

women have a vagina and are feminine." While conceptualizing gender in this binary way is less complicated, it doesn't reflect reality. We now have a better understanding of how people view themselves, and it turns out to be much more nuanced than previously understood. People are now better able to express gender in ways that are true to themselves.

Each of us is exposed to society's changing ideas about gender to differing degrees through the media, our own communities, and in our own family. Although we may not be aware of the people in our community with an identity that falls outside the binary view of gender, we can still make the effort to use inclusive language. Using new terms can be hard and feel very awkward at first. To help you, we have provided examples of inclusive, nongendered language throughout the book.

The theoretical concepts associated with gender and sexual identity are complex and multilayered. Cultural and familial ideas about gender and sexual identity influence a person's lived experience within their body, relationships, and society (Spiel et al., 2016). The learning that leads to these lived experiences begins at birth and is already ingrained by the time a child is 5 years old. These first 5 years lay the groundwork for a person's entire lifetime of learning and understanding themselves and their sexuality. These first 5 years are the jumping-off point for how to navigate through a gendered world and generally create the foundation for how one fits, or doesn't fit, in the world (Marshall & Shibazaki, 2020).

Understanding the larger theoretical concepts associated with gender and sexual orientation provides parents and other caregivers with a context for why choices like clothing, toys, and books matter for their child. Because our cultural understanding of sexuality and gender is developing so rapidly, most parents and caregivers will have had a very different set of experiences than their children will have. This chapter is designed to get you up to speed on these concepts and

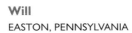

Will
EASTON, PENNSYLVANIA

Father to two children
Age when first child was born: 30

Today I've been thinking about, years ago, when Connor was playing with Johnathan's daughter. As adults were watching them getting along so well, someone said, "Maybe they'll get married someday." I have never understood why adults say such things. Our assumptions and expectations of heterosexuality seem to be hardwired, but what is the purpose of envisioning the future sexual identities of toddlers? I must have been looking for trouble when I responded, "Maybe, assuming they are both heterosexual." (This was before same-gender marriage was legal.) You could hear a pin drop after that.

Assuming sexual orientation or gender identity and expression doesn't make sense to me. Both my boys enthusiastically watched *My Little Pony* and had toys that are more traditionally for girls without any objection from us. Of greater concern was dealing with other parents or family members who might express alarm or silently disapprove. In fact, the only time I can remember trying to enforce a traditional gender script was last week. I had taken Connor shopping for some dorm supplies during a parent–child weekend at his college, and he confided that he was sweating too much. We examined the strength of antiperspirants, and he was thinking about giving the brand Secret a try. I don't know if this is still their tagline, but when I was growing up, it was: "Strong enough for a man, but made for a woman." I immediately objected, fearing ridicule from his roommate. Connor looked at me like I was from a different planet and then put the stick of Secret in the shopping basket. My earlier lessons had stuck, even if I had forgotten them.

to prepare you for the influence they will have on your child's life, both now and in the future.

The terminology used for both gender and sexual orientation varies widely by community and changes over time. At the time of writing this book (2022), we have worked to incorporate terms that are accurate and affirming. For the most current terms, you can refer to credible organizations, such as UN|HUSHED (see https://unhushed.org), GLAAD (see https://www.glaad.org), PFLAG (see https://pflag.org), or the National Center for Transgender Equality (see https://transequality.org). Likewise, having an open conversation with someone about the terms they prefer can be helpful and enlightening when such a conversation is appropriate.

As you read on, consider that there is no single right way to teach your child about gender or sexual orientation, either their own or other people's. In this chapter and the following chapters that provide age-specific support, we discuss some of the different approaches you can take to teach about these topics. In the end, you will choose what is right for your family.

GENDER

A person's *gender* comprises three parts: their biological sex, their gender identity, and their gender expression. In this section, we help you to understand these three aspects of gender and some of the differences among them. First, though, take a look at the following figure called *What's Your Gender?*, which provides some basic information on each of these three parts.

Biological Sex

Biological sex is what most people think they are talking about when they ask a soon-to-be parent the question, "Are you having a boy or a girl?" The simplicity of this question, however, belies the

What's Your Gender?

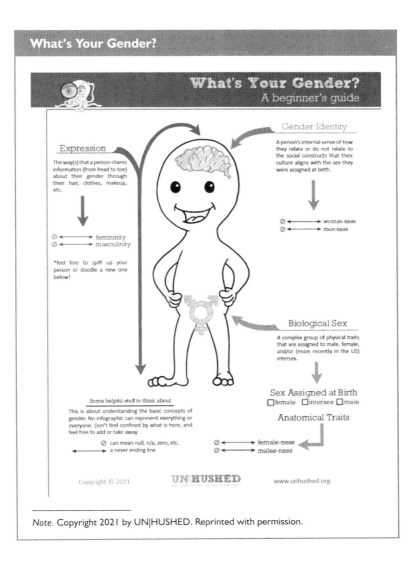

Note. Copyright 2021 by UN|HUSHED. Reprinted with permission.

complexities associated with biological sex. The details of biological sex, including the ways that it is not actually a binary construct, are considered in some depth in the Biological Sex and the Binary section in Chapter 3. If you haven't read that section recently, head back a few pages for a quick refresh.

The mechanics of biological sex don't have to be part of your daily dialogue, but you do need to proactively teach your child about genitals—their own and those of people different from them. A young child needs to be able to use terms, such as *penis*, *scrotum*, and *vulva* accurately. We also need to be able to answer their questions with honest, age-appropriate information. Over time, the language and ideas you can teach your child will become more complex. We offer a more complete outline of the mechanics of biological sex in Chapter 3.

Gender Identity

A person's *gender identity* refers to what their brain tells them about their gender and how those elements fit or don't fit with what their culture tells them about gender. The two most well-known gender identities are girl (or woman) and boy (or man). Historically, Western cultures have said that people with mostly female biological patterns are always girls or women, and people with mostly male biological patterns are always boys or men. Most parents have a look at their newborn's external genitals and make assumptions about their lifelong gender identity. While this assumption holds true for most people, it is not true for everyone. More young people understand their own identities outside of this biology-based gender binary. When parents are prepared to raise their child in a world that is not based on a gender binary, that preparation supports their child's capacity to explore and strengthen their lifelong parent–child relationship.

When a person's gender identity is what their culture assumes it is, based on their biology, that person is referred to as *cisgender*.

(This is how most people identify.) When a person's identity is other than what their culture assumes, that person is often described as *transgender*. (Fewer people identify this way, but more younger people than older people identify as noncisgender.) Importantly, gender identity is not something to assign to someone else; rather, it is something people identify for themselves. For example, some people who do not feel like either a woman or a man use words like *agender*, *gender neutral*, *gender fluid*, or *genderqueer* to describe their gender. Gender identities are often closely tied to pronouns (she/her/hers, he/him/his, they/them/theirs, and others). If using they/them/theirs with individual people is a struggle for you, the I Heart the Singular They website has some great resources (see https://iheartsingularthey.com).

Children are usually assigned a gender along with their sex. When a female child is born, families typically refer to her as a *girl*. When a male child is born, he is referred to as a *boy*. Families vary widely in terms of the degree to which they "gender" their child. Some examples of gendering a child include providing only feminine- or only masculine-associated clothing, colors, toys, and attributes to a child. For example, only offering pink or other pastel colors to a girl; providing her with only dolls and small-motor skill toys; reminding her to be soft, gentle, and kind; and commenting on how pretty she looks. For a boy, this would be only offering blue, red, or green; providing him with only trucks and large-motor skill toys; reminding him to be tough, saying men don't cry; and commenting on how strong he is. It's best to give children toys and clothing from the full spectrum of colors, both feminine and masculine, and take their lead on what they prefer—whether it's gender typical or gender atypical (Weisgram & Dinella, 2018).

Parental use of pronouns almost always ascribes a gender to newborns, even for parents who choose less gender-specific parenting. Recently, some parents have chosen to forgo she/her or he/him pronouns, using entirely they/them/their pronouns until the child is old enough to state their gender identity. There is no current research on the long-term impact of this approach. That said, the research is clear when it comes to the importance of supporting children of all ages regarding their gender identity, gender expression, and sexual orientation. Youth who experience parental and family rejection with regard to their gender or sexual orientation are at significantly greater risk of negative mental health outcomes, such as anxiety, depression, and suicide as well as an increased risk of other medical problems (Katz-Wise et al., 2016).

Gender Expression

Gender expression refers to feminine, masculine, and androgynous or gender nonconforming aspects of one's appearance, attributes, and behavior. Gender expression is the way in which we convey our gender identity to others. Gender can be expressed in the way we dress and style our hair or in our personal physical demeanor. Parents generally choose the gender expression for infants and toddlers. This often begins to shift to the child's own choices as they grow in their ability to communicate their expression preferences. For some children, this happens as young as age 2 or 3 years.

A person's gender identity is not always clear from their gender expression. Most people whose gender expression is not clearly feminine or masculine are used to answering questions about their identities. However, unless you know a person well or have a specific cause to need to know their gender identity (e.g., as a teacher might for a child in their classroom), it is generally unnecessary to ask about a person's gender. The way to ask about a person's gender, should it be useful for you to know, can be easily done by asking, "What are your preferred pronouns?"

As parents, we need to consider our views on gender and how we want to convey them to our child. We also need to think about our expectations of our child and how we want to respond if they don't conform to those expectations. While this is a personal decision for each family, there may be benefits to encouraging both feminine and masculine gender expression in every child. For instance, Sandra Bem's research found that children who incorporate both feminine and masculine elements into their identities and expressions are typically happier and have a greater degree of emotional health than children with highly gendered expressions (e.g., Bem, 1983; Bukowski et al., 2017).

The following table offers a side-by-side look at the three parts of a person's gender—biological sex, gender identity, and gender expression—and what each means.

Gender

Biological sex	Gender identity	Gender expression
An interplay of external genitalia, internal reproductive anatomy, chromosomes, hormones, and secondary sexual characteristics	An internal sense of how people do or do not relate to the sex they were assigned at birth	The gendered aspects of one's appearance, attributes, and behavior; how people visually convey themselves to others
Terminology: Female, intersex, male	Terminology: Agender, cisgender, gender-neutral, man, woman, (and others)	Terminology: Androgynous, feminine, gender nonconforming, masculine, (and others)

What you can say:

- "I love your favorite color too!"
- "Anyone can have short or long hair. It doesn't matter if they're a girl or a boy or nonbinary."
- "Your teacher uses they/them pronouns, which could be funny because we don't know anyone else who does that. Let's practice talking about them and using their pronouns."

Melissa
ASHEVILLE, NORTH CAROLINA

Mother to two children
Age when first child was born: 29

Yesterday, some boys asked River why he was wearing nail polish if he's "really a boy." River just said, "Because I like it!" They tried to say nail polish is only for girls, and he just said, "No, it's not. Anyone can wear anything they want!" The boys didn't really have a comeback for that and moved on. I felt so proud of him when he told me that story.

It has been beautiful to watch River's unique self-expression blossom over the years and to feel his confidence in himself even at 7 1/2 years old now. I've been thinking a lot about this. As soon as he could talk, he told me he wanted to have two long braids like mine—and as soon as his hair was long enough, I was happy to braid it for him. His hair is now almost as long as mine, and I still enjoy French braiding it weekly. He gets mad if anyone asks if he wants to cut it and refuses to wear it any other way, saying, "No way! Then I won't look good!" (And it's true: His hair is gorgeous!)

When he was little, he didn't care about clothing at all and often just wanted to be naked as much as possible. I mostly kept him in "gender-neutral" clothing but later realized that basically meant "boy" clothing . . . which mostly wasn't very interesting. I remember the time, around age 3, he started to notice clothes more, and he absolutely lit up when he saw bright, colorful, fun clothing: rainbows, hearts, sparkles, reversible sequins, unicorns, shiny jewelry, tutu dresses that twirl when he spins. . . . And so, I started shopping in the "girl" section, and we suddenly had no more issues with getting him dressed! (Oh, how I resent that clothes are divided into "boy" and "girl" sections and the stereotypes they each perpetuate!)

When I first took him shoe shopping, he ran straight to the "girl" section and found shiny, teal, patent leather Mary Janes that he put on immediately to wear as "tap shoes" and then insisted on wearing them out so he could dance down the street. He also picked out silver and pink tennis shoes (as he needed something practical for his outdoor preschool), and sparkly rainbow rain boots. He never gave a second look at any of the shoes in the "boy" section (which, to be fair, didn't look as fun). He still prefers "girl" shoes, and I'm quite happy with him picking what he likes—as long as they're suitable for a given activity!

People often think he's a girl because of his long braids and clothes, but he corrects them as needed or sometimes looks to me to correct them. (But he's also okay with letting it go if it's a random stranger comment and not a longer conversation.) Lately, we've gotten a lot of "what beautiful daughters" comments because he loves to have matching clothes with his baby sister, and people do a double take when I reply about what an awesome brother he is. He's very clear that he feels like a boy and that all clothing should be for whichever people like it. He thinks it's absurd for some colors or styles to be for one gender or another, and he's happy to educate anyone who questions it.

In general, we have been really lucky. I'm so grateful for our inclusive preschool that focused on kindness and affirmed kids in their choices of gender identity and expression so that he and the other kids felt safe to be themselves there.

Billie
DAVIS, CALIFORNIA

Aunt and coparent to two children
Age when first became a coparent: 35

Today, I brought the kids home, and Mia and her friend, Gemma, immediately went to play with all the toys they had strewn all over the place: blocks, books, dolls, and games on the iPad. There were a bunch of plastic dinosaur figurines and Hot Wheels cars and Mia's Barbies. Alexander plopped himself down at the end of the coffee table and looked distraught. "What's up, buddy?" I asked him. He shrugged and grabbed the Barbie. "I want to play with the doll," he said. I have never seen him struggle with what he should or shouldn't play with. Usually, the problem is getting them to clean up their toys, work on homework, or sit down long enough to have dinner . . . not whether or not they're allowed to play with a certain toy.

"So, play with the Barbie then," I said. "I can't," he replied. The girls were nearby playing with the trucks. "And why can't you?" His voice sounded more distraught and even, sweetly, younger and more innocent, "Because I'm a boy, and boys don't play with dolls." Oh, my heart. It felt like this comment came out of nowhere; it was hard to pin down where he could even have gotten that feeling or thought from . . . school, maybe? Comments from television? I've been thinking about how children today are often allowed to be who they are without any of the gender social constructs, but that was clearly an oversight.

"Oh, sweetie. Of course, you can play with dolls if you want." "Even if I'm a boy?" But before I could answer, Mia's friend, Gemma, started to laugh. "But that's so strange!" And, of course, that comment must have been one of so many comments over the course of days or weeks or even months to trickle down into his head. "Do you need to be only a boy to play with trucks?" I asked Mia and Gemma. "No," they laughed. Alexander started to smile and lighten up a bit. "You don't have to be only a boy or a girl to play with certain toys. Boys can play with dolls, and girls can play with trucks." Alexander held the doll and grabbed a toy truck and a plastic dinosaur figurine. "Is it weird?" he asked. These are the moments that stick with children, right? The pressure to not say the wrong thing was really intense, but I did the best I could:

> You know, some people may say it's weird or strange. Gemma thought it was weird. But what's important is if you listen to what makes you happy. Alexander, if you like playing with dolls, that is perfectly okay. Mia, if you want to play with trucks, that is also okay. Now you both have more toys to share with one another!

Gemma didn't say anything . . . she seemed harder to crack. But Alexander relaxed a bit, perhaps from not feeling conflicted or guilty. How intense that feeling must be at only 4 years old without the language to understand the concept of desire or gender identity. But I was so glad to see he kept playing with the doll.

SEXUAL ORIENTATION

A person's *sexual orientation* is a complex interaction of pieces: their attraction patterns, their sexual identity, and their behavior. Before we discuss each of these terms in detail, they are defined in the figure called *What's Your Sexual Orientation?*

Attraction

A conversation about sexual orientation is often based in assumptions about romantic and sexual attraction. Each of us has our own individual differences in what we find (or do not find) romantically and sexually attractive in a person. However, attraction can also be based on a wide range of other elements. For example, attraction can be about artistic skill, cognition, humor, kindness, physical bodies, religion, and so much more.

What's Your Sexual Orientation?

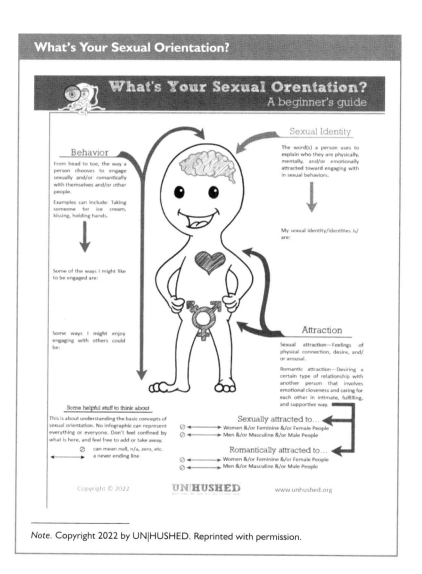

Most young children aren't yet prepared to talk (or learn) about sexual or romantic attraction. This includes adults joking about their having girlfriends or boyfriends. However, by the time children are 5 years old, they are very ready to talk (and learn) about why they choose certain people as friends and what friendship is (Carter, 2021; Papadopoulou, 2016). These are the beginning conversations that will lead to family conversations about sexual and romantic attraction over time.

Maya

AMSTERDAM, THE NETHERLANDS

Mother to one child
Age when child was born: 41

I'm still laughing at the hilarious thing Chloe did today. She's been feeling really big and proud of the fact that she's wearing underwear now instead of diapers. So, this morning, there were a bunch of workers here again, fixing the last details on the house. The hallway needed one more layer of paint, and this new, different painter showed up. Chloe usually ignores the workers, but this painter guy was quite good looking. Young and handsome and hip—different from the other workers who have been in the house whom Chloe always ignores.

Today, though, she was watching the handsome one as soon as he came through the door. She then went over to where he was working and started chatting to him. When he responded to some of her questions about what he was doing, she all of a sudden lifted up her skirt and with a tilted head and cute smile told him, "Look! I'm wearing underwear!" It made Mike and me look at each other and laugh and say, "She is probably not a lesbian." Of course, one can never be certain, but this was the clearest, but most innocent flirt I have ever seen.

Sexual Identity

A person's *sexual identity* refers to their own understanding of their attraction patterns and behavior and how those elements fit with the language their culture offers them about romantic/aromantic/sexual/asexual relationships. The acronym *LGBTQ+* (lesbian, gay, bisexual, transgender, questioning, and others) refers to some of the terms that a person might identify with, although definitely not all of them. There are myriad other terms to describe one's orientation, including the umbrella term *queer*, which includes bisexuality, pansexuality, omnisexuality, and many others.

A person's sexual identity is something they use to describe themselves, either privately or publicly. It is never something to ascribe to another person until they choose to share their identity with you. It is also never something to share about another person without their permission. Having an open conversation with someone about the terms they prefer can be helpful and enlightening when a conversation is appropriate.

Young children do not want or need language to describe their own sexual identity because they have yet to develop it for themselves. They do, however, need language to understand other people's sexual identities. It can be easier to discuss sexual identity with your child when they interact with families that include different identities. Books or other media are also great teaching tools (we provide some recommendations for you in Part II of this book).

Behavior

Sexual behavior refers to sexual and romantic behaviors between people. While examples that often come to mind for adults include vaginal, anal, and oral sex, there are many others! For example, date nights, holding hands, and dancing can all be examples of both romantic and sexual behaviors for different people. Expanding the

Judith

AMSTERDAM, THE NETHERLANDS

Mother to two children
Age when first child was born: 22

Yesterday I found out that someone famous has his son in Juno's school. He and his husband are advocates for equal love, and they share parenthood with a woman, so their kids have two fathers and a mom. I love that Juno now has the opportunity to learn about different kinds of families from actual people instead of just reading about it in a book. Now she can see with her own eyes that they are just as normal, happy, and kind as everyone else.

possibilities of what is sexual and what is romantic is often useful to support couples looking to more thoroughly enjoy their romantic and sexual relationship.

Even young children need explanations of things like the ways that kissing is different for adults in relationships and the ways that they are invited to kiss someone. Being able to talk about these things without expressing that anyone is doing anything wrong helps young children feel secure in the ways that they kiss, hug, and otherwise show appropriate affection for the people who they love.

What you can say:

- "You know how many parents you have and who they are—and your friends might have different numbers or kinds of parents. Like, some friends might have a mom and a dad, while others have a mom and a grandmother, or two dads or two moms, or only one parent who isn't a mom or a dad. Families can be all kinds of different ways!"
- "Who someone marries is up to them!"
- "Yep, you can marry a prince or a princess if they want to marry you too!"

The table that follows presents the different pieces that interact to compose a person's sexual orientation.

Sexual Orientation		
Attraction	**Sexual identity**	**Sexual behavior**
What a person finds sexually and romantically attractive or unattractive in other people	A person's understanding of their attraction to others and their sexual behavior	The sexual and romantic behaviors people choose to engage in by themselves or with other people
Includes biological sex, gender identity, gender expression, sexual identity, and more	Terminology: Asexual, bisexual, gay, lesbian, omnisexual, pansexual, queer, questioning, transgender, (and others)	Examples: Dancing, holding hands, kissing, making romantic gestures, engaging in sex

Allegra
BROOKLYN PARK, MINNESOTA

Mother to two children
Age when first child was born: 29

Today, I got the dreaded call: the one from preschool. I was busy at work when I saw the school show up on my caller ID. I picked up the phone, ready to race to school to pick up a feverish, or worse—puking!—kid. Instead, I got this.

Classroom Teacher: So, Stella had quite an interesting day today.

   Me: Oh? What do you mean by "interesting"? [I mean, being from the Midwest, "interesting" rarely means a good thing.]

Teacher: Well, first she hosted a rather nontraditional wedding with the dolls in the play corner.

   Me: Go on. . . .

Teacher: Belle and Mulan were the brides, and there were no grooms because "the princesses don't need them." And then, one of the other children, who is about to be a flower girl in a wedding this weekend, came and told me that Stella told her to tell her aunt that "she doesn't have to marry a man just because he's around. She can get married to a woman too." This child asked if I could call her aunt and let her know because "time is running out before the wedding." I love Stella's open-minded ways, but just wanted you to be aware in case any parents complain to us.

   Me: Thank you. I have to say I am impressed with Stella and glad she is paying attention to the news in the world and the way my husband and I are raising her to think about love. I will chat with her when I pick her up.

Well, when I picked her up from school today, I asked her about the doll wedding. She's only 4, but she is so smart! She told me that Belle likes to read, and Mulan saved China, and if they marry princes, they'll have to spend their days in dresses in the castle instead of learning and being awesome. Marrying each other is the best option. (I might have snorted out a bit of Diet Coke when she told me this.)

The kicker, though, is when I asked about the other child in class, and this was Stella's response: "Mommy, I had to tell her. Her aunt is an adult and maybe doesn't know all the important things. I wanted to make sure she knew all her options!"

Never a dull moment raising these firecrackers.

SUMMARY

- A person's gender is made up of their biology, gender identity, and gender expression. Someone can choose their gender expression but not their biology or identity. A young child may begin to experience and share these elements of themselves but will continue to expand them through childhood and into adolescence and even adulthood.
- A person's sexual orientation is made up of their attraction patterns, sexual identity, and sexual behaviors. Young children may begin to express these elements of themselves, like sharing that they love or want to kiss or marry a friend at school. Most young children do not do this. As a parent, it's most important to be open to whatever impulse your child expresses to you.

RESOURCES FOR PARENTS

- *The Gender Creative Child: Pathways for Nurturing and Supporting Children Who Live Outside Gender Boxes* by Diane Ehrensaft (The Experiment)
- *Trans+: Love, Sex, Romance, and Being You* by Kathryn Gonzales and Karen Rayne (Magination Press)
- *Where's MY Book?: A Guide for Transgender and Gender Non-Conforming Youth, Their Parents, & Everyone Else* by Linda Gromko (Bainbridge Books)

Chapter 5
Child Sexual Abuse:
Prevention and Response

This chapter is one of the more difficult ones to read. Take your time as you read it, especially if this is a topic that you know is triggering for you. Set up safeguards for your own emotional well-being. For example, you may choose to read this chapter when a friend or your coparent is around to help you think through and process what the information means to you and your family.

Child sexual abuse (CSA) is one of the things most parents fear most. This fear guides many parents' choices about where and with whom their children may engage over many years of their lives. This is particularly true for parents who experienced CSA themselves. Such a parental reaction is fully understandable. CSA can come with long-range, far-reaching negative effects on children's physical, psychological, interpersonal, and behavioral well-being. Experiencing CSA may be particularly harmful when a child does not have adults in their life who believe them and support them in responding to the situation. Conversely, long-lasting harmful effects resulting from CSA can sometimes be avoided if the situation is handled well.

Preventing and responding to CSA is a complex process that cannot rely exclusively on immediate family. CSA is a whole-society problem. The most effective prevention measures against your child's experiencing sexual abuse are for you to (a) provide them with comprehensive sexuality education starting in early childhood and (b) situate yourself and your family within a community that takes steps to ensure the safety of children. (Note that this strategy is different from trying to withdraw from communities because of fear of them [Martinello, 2020].)

If you are an adult who has been sexually abused, you may know the pain that comes as a result of experiencing CSA, particularly without a strong and responsible adult community. Keeping your child from having the same harmful experiences can become a focus for adult survivors of CSA. One of the best things you can do to help your child is to take care of your own healing first, just as when on an airplane, you have to secure your oxygen first before ensuring that your child gets oxygen too (Mendelson & Letourneau, 2015). Begin by knowing that it was not your fault and that help is available: places for treatment and healing and therapists who specialize in working with adult survivors of CSA. If you are near the beginning of your journey toward healing and are looking for someone to help and support you, you can speak with someone at the National Sexual Assault Hotline who is trained to help. Call 800-656-HOPE (800-656-4673) or chat online (go to https://hotline.rainn.org/online).

In this chapter, we help you to understand CSA, including how it is defined, typical abuser characteristics, and common traits of victimization. We then discuss ways to help prevent CSA, how to recognize the signs when it does happen, and how to find help for children who have been harmed by CSA.

DEFINITION OF CHILDHOOD SEXUAL ABUSE

Unfortunately, defining CSA is not a simple matter. Even organizations like the American Professional Society on the Abuse of Children (APSAC) and the World Health Organization (WHO) differ in the extent of their definitions (Klika & Conte, 2017; WHO, 1999).

APSAC, for example, explicitly includes both touching and non-touching abuse and provides detailed examples, whereas the WHO definition is less detailed and acknowledges societal differences in laws and taboos. Some elements remain consistent across various definitions:

- CSA involves a child under 18.
- CSA involves sexual contact but can include touching, non-touching, or both.
- The child is either unable to consent or unable to understand the implications of the sexual contact.
- The abuser has more power than the child because of the abuser's age, size, cognitive ability, or social standing.
- A child can exhibit problematic sexual behaviors that harm another child.

Many people wonder about the prevalence of CSA. How common is it? This is also a difficult question to answer. Because researchers use different definitions and different methods for gathering data, the statistics we get as a result vary widely. The best and most recent analysis, which combines data across many studies, shows that about one in 10 children are sexually abused (Sedlak et al., 2010; Townsend & Rheingold, 2013). We know, however, that all forms of family abuse have increased during COVID-19 lockdowns. The data we have now are from before COVID, and it remains to be seen if post-COVID numbers will return to pre-COVID levels.

TYPICAL CHARACTERISTICS OF ABUSERS

Adults who sexually abuse are typically friendly people a child already has contact with through their family, school, or other integrated community in their life. *The vast majority of abusers are a person known to both the child and parent(s).* Working to prevent CSA is not the same as teaching your child "beware of strangers." Although a sexual abuser may have been sexually abused as a child themselves, they also may not have been. They are less likely to be actually attracted to children and more likely to be abusive for a wide range of reasons, including anger, intimacy problems, loneliness, hypersexuality, a desire for power and control, and more.

Approximately one third of abused children are hurt by other children. Children who exhibit problematic sexual behaviors are typically much more impulse driven and random when compared with adult abusers. Their sexual behavior may be born out of a misunderstanding of appropriate boundaries between themselves and someone who is younger, smaller, or less able to understand the context of sexual activity. Youth abusers may or may not have been abused themselves, and the vast majority of them *do not* become systemic abusers as they grow into adults. While the overwhelming majority of adult abusers are men, abusers who are children are more evenly split between girls and boys.

COMMON PATTERNS OF VICTIMIZATION

CSA by adults is typically (although not always) an orchestrated process whereby the perpetrator builds a relationship with the child slowly over time. Abusers work to fulfill the needs and desires of a child, such as giving gifts like candy or toys or giving the child needed attention. They then use small, inappropriate behaviors or touches to see how the child responds and whether they will tell a trusted adult or keep the behavior secret. Abusers purposely check to see if an adult will set a boundary. This friendship-building process is called *grooming*. Once a friendship is solidified, abusers escalate their behavior.

While *every child is vulnerable to CSA*, there are some particular risk factors. Children who do not have information about bodies,

Maya

AMSTERDAM, THE NETHERLANDS

Mother to one child
Age when child was born: 41

I came home from an errand yesterday and found Chloe and Mike snuggling together in bed. Chloe had just come out of the bath, and she was naked, while Mike was not. They were snuggling under the covers because she had gotten cold while drying off, and it really freaked me out. I told Chloe to get dressed and told Mike that I thought that this was really unhealthy and not right. Then Mike got really angry with me for thinking that he would ever do anything inappropriate to Chloe and for not trusting him with his own daughter. So, it turned into a big fight.

I don't know if Mike was right, or if I was. I do know that I'm extra sensitive about boundaries with Chloe because there was sexual abuse in my dad's side of the family. Even before the abuse came out into the open (was I 8? 9 years old?), I think the family history of abuse influenced Dad on a subconscious level—like in the way he wasn't able to be physically close with us kids in a healthy way, and that also impacted me. So now, when I see Chloe and Mike together in certain ways, it's such a trigger for me. I have such strong feelings around unhealthy physical intimacy between fathers and daughters, and I wonder if I'm even totally off sometimes because of my background. I do know that my sensitivity has definitely led to tension, misunderstandings, and arguments between Mike and me about Chloe and what seems to me to be inappropriate intimacy. But then, of course, maybe it's not inappropriate. I don't know.

body safety, and sexual development (the information in Part II of this book) are at higher risk for abuse. Abusers also target children who have fewer protective features in their home life, such as children who have parents who aren't around as much or children who are lonely, depressed, or separated from a strong community. Children who live with stepparents or single parents are at greater risk.

Other major factors of abuse are gender and disabilities. Females are 5 times more likely to be abused than males. Intellectually or physically disabled children are about 4 times as likely to be victims of CSA. Intellectually or physically disabled children can and should learn about sexuality and body safety.

WAYS TO HELP PREVENT CHILD SEXUAL ABUSE

Prevention is a critical component of reducing CSA and is substantially more impactful than responding after abuse has begun. It involves teaching boundaries, encouraging open conversations with a wide range of adults, and implementing other protective factors that prevent a child from being seen as vulnerable by a problematic adult (Rudolph et al., 2018).

Teaching Boundaries and Consent

Boundary setting is an essential aspect of sexuality, and children are learning about it all the time. If you have a young child who is old enough to be moving around the house on their own, you are very familiar with boundary setting in general. Whether you have baby gates up, are reminding a toddler that we use gentle touch instead of hitting, or are explaining to your kindergartner yet again why they cannot have more Halloween candy before dinner, parenting involves *a lot* of teaching about boundaries.

In this chapter, we discuss the physical boundaries we need to teach to keep our child safer. Whether or not we are discussing boundaries per se, we have spoken or unspoken rules about who can be touched where, when, and how. We want to raise young people who can confidently say no and who respect others when they do the same.

It's important to be intentional about teaching boundaries for several reasons. When kids are aware of their boundaries and know that their boundaries should be respected, they feel more empowered to set limits with others. Children should know that their body is theirs and that they get to decide what kind of physical interaction

Florence
AMSTERDAM, THE NETHERLANDS

Mother to two children
Age when first child was born: 40

Early on, I taught my child that he has the right to choose who touches him and how. I feel very strongly about the importance of teaching him these boundaries. Sometimes that was hard for me, though, like when my little 4-year-old didn't want kisses—for years! (As he got older, he figured out the ways he was comfortable with kisses.)

The fact that he knew he had ownership over his own body also became a way he would assert control in different situations. When it was time to put on pajamas, for example, if he didn't want to do it, he would say, "It's my body!" I found this hilarious and totally acceptable. My coparent did not. Then it was my job to figure out what my boundaries were. (In that case, he could wear whatever he wanted to wear to bed as long as it was clean.) Now that he's older, he is better able to understand the nuances of boundaries and that he has control over how he's touched, but he still has to do the nonnegotiable things we ask him to do.

is good for them. Explicitly teaching about personal boundaries can also help keep children safer from sexual abuse. They will know that unwanted touching is inappropriate and that they can talk with you if they experience anything that makes them feel uncomfortable.

GENITALS

The first thing we parents might think of when teaching kids about sexual boundaries is who does and does not get to touch their genitals. This can be tricky because we want to teach children that their genitals are special and often private without instilling shame or stigma around them. We need to teach kids that genitals are different from other parts of the body. They are wonderful and special. They are just as normal as the rest of the body. And they are different because we only want people touching or looking at them in particular circumstances.

When your child is an infant and young toddler, they have a more limited range of caregivers. This is the time to focus on emphasizing how wonderful their *whole* body is, including genitals. You can begin by acknowledging that genitals are interesting and touching them feels good; teaching your child the names of the different parts of their genitals; and showing them that bodily functions like peeing, pooping, and farting are normal. As they become more verbal, we need to inform them that only certain people get to touch their genitals: themselves; parents or other primary caregivers in very specific situations; or doctors, when another trusted adult is present.

NUDITY

Views on child nudity, both in private and public, can vary widely from person to person and within the same family. Child nudity is not a known risk factor for CSA in itself. CSA offenders find ways to be around children they can get close to whether at a day care,

Maya

AMSTERDAM, THE NETHERLANDS

Mother to one child
Age when child was born: 41

Chloe, Mike, and I were hanging out this afternoon. Chloe likes to take off her clothes when she is at home, so she was in just a tank top and no underwear. Mike was playing some tickling game with her like he has been doing from time to time since she was a baby. Now that she is 3, he still plays with her that way. He was blowing behind her ear to make her laugh and tickling her sides and stuff. She was laughing while saying "Stop" but also instructing him to do more, saying things like, "Now tickle me here, blow here, or kiss me here!" (He has grown a bit of a beard, so that was extra ticklish, I guess). And he was doing just as instructed by her, thinking it was super cute.

Then, in this same innocent exchange, she told him all of a sudden, "Now kiss me here!" and pointed to her vulva. He seemed taken aback and told her he couldn't do that. It made me uncomfortable also, and I jumped in immediately saying, "No, no, that's not for other people to touch!" Our responses seemed to really confuse her. "Why not?" she asked. And she actually pleaded for quite some time, "Please, please, Daddy, kiss me there. It would feel funny!" It seemed she couldn't really understand why sensitive places like her sides and the back of her ears are all right for tickles and kisses, but her vulva, which is also very sensitive, would not be.

an after-school program, or at home. Whatever the comfort level with nudity in your own family, you can teach important messages about safety to your child. In addition to earlier messages about genitals, children need to learn that nudity is, or is not, appropriate in different situations. Even if your child is used to being naked at home or at play dates in the kiddie pool, for instance, it isn't appropriate to take off their clothes at school or the grocery store.

Parental attitudes and cultural norms have the greatest influence on how children themselves feel about nudity. Many children love to be naked and take their clothes off whenever they are allowed. Around 3 or 4 years of age, kids become more aware of what is considered public or private. As they get older, children will naturally become more self-conscious about being naked in front of other people. We parents usually see feelings like embarrassment and self-consciousness crop up around ages 5 or 6. This is the same time when many children start to be conscious about nudity and might want more privacy for themselves when it comes to being naked.

Specific family rules about nudity are less important than attitudes about the body. In your family, how do you encourage your child to feel comfort and pride in their body? How do you foster appreciation for bodies that are different from theirs? The answers to those questions can involve being naked around each other, or not. The one rule we—Laura and Karen—think it's important to adhere to is this: If a child ever expresses discomfort or desire for themselves or others in the family not to be naked, their wishes should be respected.

Rules around nudity are a time when we parents can see the influence of gender stereotypes. Some people's comfort with nakedness depends on the child's gender and often leans toward being more restrictive for girls. Girls are reported to be victims of CSA more frequently than boys. As a result, teaching children different rules about nudity based on gender may feel protective to some. However, this approach shames girls about their body and tells them that boys can be more physically free. Moreover, boys are also victims of CSA. We want to offer all children the same level of protection and also teach them equally about the joys of their body.

AFFECTION

Kids need to know that they get to decide when and with whom to be affectionate. Your child might be gregarious and affectionate with everyone. And that's perfectly okay. If your child is wary of people they don't know well, that's also very normal. Yet, there are many situations in which children are asked to be affectionate even when they don't feel like it. Consider a visit with a relative, for example. Many times, children are told, "Give Auntie a hug." When they hesitate, they are told more insistently: "Come on, now. You remember Auntie!" Even if they do remember Auntie, if they don't feel comfortable giving and getting a hug from her, they shouldn't have to do that.

Asking someone to respect a child's choice to be hugged, kissed, picked up, or held on someone's lap can offend some adults, especially family members. Some parents also feel that it reflects poorly on them, as though they are not teaching their children to be polite and respect family or elders. Respecting your child's boundaries is not allowing them to be impolite. They can still be expected to greet people politely. Supporting your child when they set a boundary is a reflection of informed parenting. Explain to the adult the reasons you are modeling boundaries in this way, such as setting precedents for safety and consent, and encourage them to not take it personally. If you encounter resistance to this concept, remember that your most important job is to foster the health and happiness of your child, even if it means doing things others don't like.

Parents can also teach about boundaries by respecting boundaries ourselves. When approaching other people's kids, ask their permission before embracing them. While we might adore our best friend's child, it's okay if they don't always feel like a hug. We are happy that they are doing—or not doing—what feels safe to them. Instead, when we see kids we know and love, we can ask them if they would like a hug. If we don't get a hug or an enthusiastic yes, we ask if we can give them a high five or a fist bump instead. In the end, kids need to learn to acknowledge others by saying hello or goodbye, but they shouldn't have to be physically affectionate.

PRIVACY

Learning about privacy is a necessary part of childhood. We can work on finding a balance of supporting children's growing understanding of appropriate bodily boundaries (i.e., both their own and others' privacy) while also bolstering children in being proud of, supported in, and understanding their own bodies and those of others. Understanding what parts of the body are private or personal (depending on your language choice) varies by family, but it is important for all children to understand that some areas of the body should not be shown to others, the genitals especially.

Some families and books use the term "private parts" for genitals. Using this language has the benefit of emphasizing that genitals are only to be touched and seen in specific, more limited, circumstances. At the same time, using the term "genitals" emphasizes that there isn't anything inherently wrong with them. Genitals are a part of the body that are as important and normal as the rest of the body for which we don't use additional, slang terms. What's most important is that the language you choose feels supportive of a positive body image for you. We want you to be able to say whatever words you choose with love. For example, if you find that words like "private parts" make you think or feel a sense of shame, that's not the best choice for your family. Talk with your coparent, if you have one, about what feels like the most life-affirming language for both of you.

Whatever language you choose, explaining to your child the role that boundaries play in interacting with others can be powerful moments of connection. Have these conversations proactively while snuggling, playing, or being otherwise connected to your child so that they feel that discussions about anatomy and boundaries are healing, connecting conversations rather than ones that happen out of anger or being pushed away.

ROUGHHOUSE PLAY

Another opportunity to teach about respecting boundaries is during tickling and roughhouse play. Roughhousing or wrestling is healthy and fun when everyone enjoys it. It's good for kids and for grown-ups too. It's also a great opportunity to teach about boundaries. Establish a family rule that as soon as anyone says the words "no" or "stop," everyone stops. Even if it sounds like kids are saying it in jest—just being playful—teach them that if they express a desire to stop the activity, everyone playing will stop and check in. You can always resume the fun.

A child's nonverbal behavior that indicates a lessening of interest in physical play should also be a cue to check in. If they didn't ask for a pause in the play but seemed like they needed a break, let them know why you stopped. With tickling, for example, stop regularly, and let them catch their breath. They will certainly let you know if they want more. This also goes for siblings. Teach siblings that a person's saying "Stop!" should be respected immediately. In addition to "stop," you can also use terms like "pause" or "time-out," or just make the time-out hand gesture. Children can learn that there are all kinds of ways to say stop, including using facial expressions and body language.

Learning the Signs of Feeling Unsafe

When a person feels unsafe, their body has physiological responses. We list many of them in the chart called *Physiological Signs That We Feel Unsafe* that follows. Children can learn to recognize these signs, listen to them, and let us know if they have been in a situation that has made them feel unsafe. Educate2Empower publishing makes a useful poster to help talk about this topic (see the Resources for Kids section at the end of this chapter).

Physiological Signs That We Feel Unsafe
• Feel sick in the tummy
• Feel sweaty, such as sweaty palms or brow
• Get goosebumps
• Hair feels like it's standing on end
• Heart beats fast
• Legs feel wobbly
• Need to go to the bathroom
• Feel shaky all over
• Start to cry or feel like crying

Parents can also teach these signs during typically stressful situations when our child is with us. For example, if our child is starting preschool or school and feeling nervous, we can ask them what their body is feeling. Are they feeling sick in the tummy? Do they have to pee all of a sudden? Let your child know that if they ever feel unsafe when you aren't there, they should tell you about it so you can help. It's a great lesson in helping them listen to what their body is telling them.

Listening to Your Elders . . . Mostly

Children who are taught to obey authority without question are at higher risk for abuse. If they think they are always supposed to do what they are told, they are less likely to set boundaries when they feel unsafe.

While we parents want kids to cooperate with teachers, babysitters, grandparents, coaches, and other authority figures, they need to know that they never have to do what someone else tells them if it makes them feel unsafe or if it involves genitals. Let them know that this includes anyone: kids, adults, family members, or friends.

Talking With Trusted Adults

Kids who are abused are sometimes told they have to keep their experience a secret with their abuser. If a child is abused, we adults want to know about it so we can help them. Teach your child that they can always talk with you or another trusted adult. Brainstorm with your child about other trusted adults they can talk with if they ever need help. We understand that kids sometimes have thoughts and feelings they don't want to share, but *no one should ever tell them* to keep a secret. On the other hand, surprises are fun. Surprises are a little like secrets because we do hide them from someone. The big difference is that there is always a plan to reveal a surprise.

Moreover, explicitly tell your child repeatedly over the years that if they ever tell you about something that has happened, no matter how bad it is, you will not be angry with them and you will always keep them and yourself safe. You can show this to your child through your actions. If your child is nervous about telling you something—maybe they know they did something you will be upset about—reward them for being forthcoming. Thank them for telling you, stay calm, and avoid outbursts of frustration or anger. The trust you build is more important than whatever they did.

While we want to encourage our child to communicate, keep in mind that it is never the fault of a child if they don't divulge abuse. The abuser, whether a child or adult, is likely to be in a position of power (e.g., by being older or stronger or through their social position), and it's natural for a child not to want to talk about what's happened.

Using Books to Teach Kids About Body Safety

Books are a great way to teach kids about many aspects of sexuality, and many books are available to help teach young children important messages about body safety. You can find books on body safety in both the Resources for Parents and Resources for Kids sections at the end of this chapter.

Whenever you intend to read a book to your child about sexuality, it's helpful to read the book on your own first. That way, you can check in with your level of comfort about the topic and address your discomfort ahead of time, if that's needed. You can also make sure the book contains messages and language you agree with. Because most young children can't read yet, you can change the language of books to convey the messages and language you prefer.

Vetting Caregivers

While we can teach children body safety skills, it is ultimately our responsibility to protect children to the best of our ability. CSA offenders are cunning and very difficult to identify. Teaching your child the body safety messages we talked about earlier is a big step toward preventing it. That said, one of the best measures to prevent your child from experiencing CSA is talking with the adults in your child's life and ensuring they are trained in how to prevent and identify CSA.

It's worth it to have hard conversations with caregivers like babysitters, teachers, coaches, and others. Before you leave your child in someone's care, let them know that you teach your child about body safety, correct names for genitals, and boundaries. They should be prepared to respect your child's boundaries, whether that is in regard to hugging, tickling, or any other physical contact.

When touring a preschool, day care, or school, for example, ask questions about how they handle things like diaper changes, toilet training, naming anatomy, and sexual situations that arise. Let them know that, in your family, you use accurate names for genitalia, so teachers may hear those terms from your child. Encourage those caregivers to use accurate anatomical terms as well. In addition, ask what kinds of training their staff have had concerning preventing CSA and what policies they have in place to prevent it. Evidence-based training programs are known to help prevent and identify CSA in child care settings. If your child will be attending day care, preschool, or school, ask about their policies and see if they have or will provide a training program for their staff. It can be helpful to have resources on hand to recommend, such as from these organizations: Darkness2Light (see https://www.d2l.org) and Parenting Safe Children (see https://parentingsafechildren.com).

Judith
AMSTERDAM, THE NETHERLANDS

Mother to two children
Age when first child was born: 22

A mom I know came over today for coffee and brought her child, Francine. The mom and I were talking about bad experiences we had in school, and she told me about something that happened while Francine was at school. One of the teachers got suspended for inappropriately touching one of the kids. I know stuff like this sometimes happens, but hearing about it happening from someone so close to me got me quite scared for my own children.

I'm really terrified about this topic. I want to protect my children, but I don't want to explicitly tell them about that specific danger. I still don't really know how to deal with it. I do wonder if there is a way, a technique, that protects them but allows them to still live in their wonderful, innocent, fairy-tale world.

Having Conversations

The most effective way to prevent your child from experiencing CSA is to be a proactive, engaged caregiver who introduces conversations about sex and sexuality, including consent and boundaries, and makes them a fluent part of regular conversations. This provides your child with a defined space to talk with you openly about their comfort levels with people in their lives, any grooming behaviors that might take place, or any other concerning experiences they may have.

In their publication *Straight Talk About Child Sexual Abuse: A Prevention Guide for Parents*, the Enough Abuse Campaign recommends that parents have a series of conversations with their child about a number of topics (Bernier, 2014). In this section, we present those five conversations as stated in that prevention guide. The conversation topics, though, are interspersed with specific, concrete suggestions from us, your authors, about what you can say to your children as a means of having those conversations. You can start having these conversations by the time your child is 3 years of age.

CONVERSATION I

> All parts of our bodies are good and we can speak about them respectfully. It's best to use the right names for private parts, like penis, vagina, breasts, buttocks or butt. (Bernier, 2014, p. 7)

Authors' note: When parents say these words with confidence and a positive affect, they set the stage for their child to feel more comfortable telling them about sexually inappropriate behavior or abuse. Conversely, if you're embarrassed about genitals or about using correct terminology, you are likely to be sending the message that talking about genitals is taboo.

What you can say:

- "Your *whole* body is wonderful."
- "In our family, we use the real names for genitals like *penis*, *scrotum*, *vagina*, and *vulva*."
- "We don't have time to wait right now, so I'm going to gently move your hands so I can put your clean diaper on."
- "That's your penis/scrotum/vulva."
- "Your genitals are just for you, but I need to put a little bit of lotion on that rash. When you're older, you can do it yourself."

CONVERSATION 2

Grown-ups and older children have no business "playing" with your private body parts. Sometimes grown-ups need to help young children with washing or wiping these private parts, but that's not the same as playing with them. Sometimes doctors need to examine you. But it's never without a nurse or parent in the room, and it's never a secret. (Bernier, 2014, p. 7)

 What you can say:

- "It's okay for you to touch your own genitals, but other people shouldn't be touching or playing with them."
- "You wash your own genitals because they're only for you to touch, but sometimes I do need to help you with things like cleaning poop or if they're hurting or itching. Or sometimes if we go to the doctor, they may need to check your genitals, but I would be with you for that."

CONVERSATION 3

Grown-ups and older children never, ever need help from children with their private parts. If someone asks you for this kind of help, tell me right away, even if it's someone in our family or someone we know. If anyone shows you their private parts, pictures of private parts, or asks to take pictures of your private parts, you can tell me. I promise I will listen and not be angry.

If you ever feel "mixed up" about secrets, feelings, or private body parts, tell me and I will help you. (Bernier, 2014, p. 7)

 What you can say:

- "If other people—kids or adults—need help with their genitals, they need to get help from a grown-up and never from a kid."
- "I want to make sure you know that you can tell me anything, even if it feels embarrassing. I won't think there's anything wrong with you, and I won't be mad."
- "No one should ever show you their genitals or pictures of genitals. Those are private. It's one thing if people are in a changing room getting dressed, but that's very different from someone who is alone with you."
- "If you ever have a weird or icky feeling about something, it's good to tell your mom or me so we can help you."

Conversation 4

It's important that you do not touch anyone else's private parts. It could make them feel upset, confused, or angry and could get you in trouble. If you are wondering about these things, come tell me and we can talk about it. (Bernier, 2014, p. 7)

 What you can say:

- "Genitals are private."
- "Your genitals are just for you, and other people's genitals are just for them."
- "We don't touch other people's genitals or breasts."

Conversation 5

Surprises are fun for children but secrets are not okay. Surprises are secrets meant to be told, like a surprise party. But other secrets can be dangerous because they don't let me know if you're safe. (Bernier, 2014, p. 7)

What you can say:

- "You can tell me about anything important that happens, and I won't be mad at you."
- "I want you to know that you can always tell me things, especially things that might have been upsetting, so I can help to keep you safe."
- "If you don't feel comfortable talking to me about something, there are other people you can talk to like Aunt Bea or your teacher. Who do you feel safe talking to?"
- "If you think someone is doing something unsafe or uncomfortable, you can always tell me about it."

You will not have these conversations all at once! Rather, they will be spread out over years in ways that feel natural and connecting between you and your child.

Melissa
ASHEVILLE, NORTH CAROLINA

Mother to two children
Age when first child was born: 29

We had friends over this week, and while the mom and I were talking inside, her daughter and River went out to play on the deck. I was kind of keeping an eye on them through the sliding glass door but couldn't really hear them since they had shut it—which was fine, as they both tend to be loud.

At some point, I realized it seemed awfully quiet, and I couldn't see them. I went and slid open the door to check in, and they peered out from behind a chair, whispering to each other and laughing, and just said, "Stay out of our fort!" They seemed okay, and the other mom kept talking, so I just stayed closer to the door, where I could see better. (I know I'm kind

(continues)

(continued)

of hypervigilant about kids being alone together as they get closer to the age I was when my own sexual abuse started.)

A few minutes later, it got quiet again, and they had disappeared from view completely. As I went out to check on them, they both quickly pulled up their pants and giggled nervously. I asked what they were up to, and the girl said, "Nothing. Just playing house."

River giggled, and I asked, "Do either of you need to pee? I thought I just saw your pants down. If you need to use the bathroom, please come inside and give each other privacy." They said, "We don't need to pee! We just want to keep playing!" I got down on their level and said, "Well, if you want to keep playing out here, you need to stay where I can see you and keep your pants up, please." They kind of looked disappointed and maybe a little guilty but agreed, and we adults brought our conversation outside to be with them, and that was the end of it.

It all felt in the range of normal curiosity, but I also am not sure if we should have had a more explicit conversation, if more supervision would be needed at their play dates going forward, or if it's actually okay for them to just look at each other's differences, to get their curiosity satisfied in a safe space, but not to touch? But maybe that just happened and it's sufficient . . .?

I've heard that our childhood trauma comes up when our kids reach the age we were when it happened to us, and since mine started around 4 and they're close to that age, I'm trying to notice my triggers and pause before I respond to River's questions or naked antics. But sometimes I don't know what's appropriate, or how to respond, when my own upbringing was so very sexual that I didn't know what was age appropriate back then . . . and still don't really know now!

SIGNS OF CHILD SEXUAL ABUSE

It is not possible to prevent all CSA. If your child experiences this kind of abuse, it is not because you have failed as a parent, or because you were lacking in vigilance, or that you should have, in some way, known and been able to prevent it. Rather, you should take the steps from earlier in this chapter, watch for warning signs, and take steps toward healing if abuse does occur.

The first sign that CSA has or is occurring is usually through emotional and social changes. Some examples include

- becoming withdrawn;
- refusal, reluctance, or fear of certain people;
- regression in behavior;
- sudden increase in anger, outbursts, and other emotional distress; or
- sudden increase in nightmares or other difficulties sleeping.

Many of these warning signs can also be indications of other emotionally difficult life circumstances or potentially indications of these elements in the lives of your child's friends. If you are worried about your child or another child, based on these warning signs, reach out to a professional to help assess the child's experiences and needs.

Some kinds of sexual behavior are normal and natural, and other kinds are not. Normal behaviors for the early childhood years can include

- asking questions about sex, reproduction, and anatomy;
- being too close to another person;
- being naked;
- engaging in play that involves reproduction;
- staring at another person, including in the bathroom and when they are changing clothes;
- touching and exploring their own genitals; or
- touching another person's genitals or breasts.

Some sexual behaviors are problematic and indicate you should reach out for help in determining whether the behavior is an indication of sexual abuse. Warning signs in the early childhood years can include

- advanced sexual knowledge;
- pictures drawn of people that frequently and substantially feature genitals;
- frequent sexual play that cannot be redirected;
- repeated sexual engagement after being given boundaries;
- simulation of specific adult sex acts; or
- unusual, compulsive, angry, aggressive, or forceful play or specific sexual play.

There are also physical warning signs associated with CSA. Some examples include

- discomfort with walking or sitting,
- genital discharge, or
- unexplained genital bruising.

All of these physical issues may be explained by other elements (e.g., injury, allergic reactions), but they should all be checked out by a medical professional.

Melissa
ASHEVILLE, NORTH CAROLINA

Mother to two children
Age when first child was born: 29

We just had an intense few days of parenting. River has been in a phase where he is obsessed with his anus. If he's not wearing clothes, he'll run around the house having naked dance parties and then randomly bend over, spread his butt cheeks, and say, "Look at my anus!" I've been talking about how that's not appropriate, but he doesn't seem to care.

Well, apparently, he told his babysitter, "Sometimes Daddy sticks his finger in my anus." She tried to ask him some more questions about it (gently, curiously) and was fairly concerned, even though River didn't really have much else to say about it. So, she talked to me.

I happen to know that Steve is not at all into anal *anything*. When I brought it up with him, without saying which caregiver or teacher had said it, he was obviously genuinely surprised and said he would never do such a thing. After some reflection, he said maybe River was making it up to get a reaction.

While that's certainly possible, given the nature of this particular child (who loves to get a rise out of people!), I pointed out to Steve that, technically, one of his teachers might be mandated to report it as sexual abuse. Steve was taken aback and said, "Sexual?! There's nothing sexual about an anus!"—which does indeed tally with my experiences of him as a sexual partner and significantly alleviated my concerns.

I went back and talked to the babysitter about this conversation. She agreed it was possible that River was making it up—he couldn't really say anything else about it and said it didn't hurt (which I'm pretty sure it would, if it had really happened).

I asked River about it myself, and he didn't seem to have any concerning energy around it. So, we talked about how that is never a funny thing to joke about, but if anybody ever does touch any of his private areas (including his anus), or if anyone does anything to his body that he's uncomfortable with, he should definitely tell me first. And then we talked about the story of "The Boy Who Cried Wolf" and why it's a serious thing to not make up stuff like that because we need to be able to trust him to help keep him safe. He seemed to get it . . . I hope!

Steve and I also talked about River being ready to wipe his own butt more consistently so that this won't be an issue going forward, as he won't need Dad or anybody else touching his butt. He's still not that great at wiping, even with a wet wipe, but he's getting better. He now knows that it's his job and that his anus is also a private part that he shouldn't be joking about or showing to others. But, phew! Such a hard few days of processing!

HOW TO GET HELP IF YOUR CHILD EXPERIENCES CHILD SEXUAL ABUSE

If you see in your child any of the warning signs we've just talked about, the first thing you can do is to stay calm in front of your child. This will protect your child from becoming distressed or elevating their distress as a result of your own feelings. In addition, reach out for help. Professionals, both medical and psychological, are trained on how to engage with young children without asking leading questions and without harming the child's sense of self. Also, trust your gut. If you are worried that things are not right with your child, reach out for help.

To get support on how to find help, call the National Sexual Assault Hotline at 800-656-HOPE (800-656-4673) or chat online (go to https://hotline.rainn.org/online). Also, read through the resources listed at the end of this chapter.

HOW TO HELP CHILDREN WHO EXHIBIT PROBLEMATIC SEXUAL BEHAVIORS

Children ages 5 and under who exhibit problematic sexual behaviors need huge amounts of education, information, guidance, love, and support. They need the caregivers around them to know that they will not always necessarily exhibit problematic sexual behavior. Healing and boundaries are both possible! Children who exhibit problematic sexual behaviors are often grappling with behavior problems in many arenas, and the families will need professional guidance on managing their growth and their healing (Shawler et al., 2018). A great place to start is the National Center on the Sexual Behavior of Youth's parent corner (for more details, see the Resources for Parents section at the end of the chapter).

WHAT TO DO NOW?

Knowing about CSA and taking steps to help prevent it in your own family is critical, necessary work. However, as we discussed in the opening to this chapter, this is a systemic problem that demands systemic responses rather than just individual households. We encourage you to take a stand against CSA at the systemic level by joining the Pledge to Prevent campaign. Visit https://www.pledgetoprevent. org and become part of the movement against child sexual assault.

SUMMARY

- CSA is difficult to define. All definitions involve sexual contact with a child by someone with more power. Abusers are typically someone a child and their parent(s) already know.
- Teaching young children about boundaries, bodies, affection, connection, privacy, and what to do if they feel uncomfortable is a critical part of raising young children to be resilient against CSA. When children are part of a community of people who they trust will believe them and protect them, they are protected against CSA and have ready access to get help if they were to experience it. Having adults who believe them and help them when CSA occurs is very protective against the long-term emotional and psychological ramifications of experiencing CSA.

RESOURCES FOR PARENTS

Online

- Association for the Treatment & Prevention of Sexual Abuse: https://www.atsa.com
- Darkness to Light: https://www.d2l.org

- Enough Abuse Campaign: https://enoughabuse.org
- National Sexual Assault Hotline: 800.656.HOPE (800-656-4673) or chat online at https://hotline.rainn.org/online
- Parenting Safe Children: https://parentingsafechildren.com
- National Center on the Sexual Behavior of Youth, *Parents* webpage: https://www.ncsby.org/content/parents

Books

- *Off Limits: A Parent's Guide to Keeping Kids Safe From Sexual Abuse* by Sandy K. Wurtele and Feather Berkower (Safer Society Press)
- *Understanding Children's Sexual Behaviors: What's Natural and Healthy* by Toni Cavanagh Johnson (Neari Press)

RESOURCES FOR KIDS

You will also find these resources listed by age group in Part II.

Boundaries and Consent

- Poster titled "My Early Warning Signs" from Educate2Empower Publishing: https://e2epublishing.info/posters
- *A Hug* by Nicola Manton; Magali Garcia, Illustrator (self-published)
- *Ask First, Monkey! A Playful Introduction to Consent and Boundaries* by Juliet Clare Bell; Abigail Tompkins, Illustrator (Jessica Kingsley Publishers)
- *Can I Give You a Squish?* by Emily Neilson (Penguin Random House)
- *Everyone's Got a Bottom* by Tess Rowley; Jodi Edwards, Illustrator (Family Planning Queensland)

- *Good Pictures, Bad Pictures Jr.: A Simple Plan to Protect Young Minds* by Kristen A. Jenson; Debbie Fox, Illustrator (Glen Cove Press)
- *Miles Is the Boss of His Body* by Abbie Schiller and Samantha Kurtzman-Counter (The Mother Company)
- *My Body Sends a Signal: Helping Kids Recognize Emotions and Express Feelings* by Natalia Maguire; Anastasia Zababashkina, Illustrator (Maguire Books)
- *No Means No!* by Jayneen Sanders; Cherie Zamazing, Illustrator (Upload Publishing)
- *Uncle Willy's Tickles: A Child's Right to Say No* (2nd ed.) by Marcie Aboff; Kathleen Gartner, Illustrator (Magination Press)
- *What Lily Knows* by Jessica Smarr (UN|HUSHED)
- *Will Ladybug Hug?* by Hilary Leung (Scholastic)

Boundaries and Consent for Atypical Kids

- *An Exceptional Children's Guide to Touch: Teaching Social and Physical Boundaries to Kids* by Hunter Manasco; Katharine Manasco, Illustrator (Jessica Kingsley Publishers)

Song/Video

- Teeny Tiny Stevies, *Boss of My Own Body*, YouTube video: https://www.youtube.com/watch?v=nLpjNJnXZlU

The Ages and Stages of Teaching Sexual Health During Early Childhood

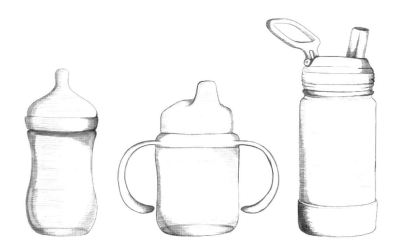

INTRODUCTION: THE AGES AND STAGES OF TEACHING SEXUAL HEALTH DURING EARLY CHILDHOOD

The ways that young children learn are myriad and build on themselves over time. This is true about sexuality, relationships, and sexual health, as it is true about every other component of development. Consider how children learn to read and write. They start by listening in utero even before they are born (May et al., 2011). Infants don't always understand our words and sentences, but they are listening nonetheless. They hear our sounds and intonations. They watch our mouths and facial expressions (Ichikawa & Yamaguchi, 2014). Early on, they begin to vocalize, trying out how their noises feel and sound. They notice how we respond.

As they grow past infancy, children begin to understand more of what we say. They can follow our instructions, for example, before they can talk. Then they say their first words and begin to quickly build a lexicon. Then sentences come. They are simple sentences at first and then build to more complicated ones. Next, they learn their ABCs. By the time they are at the end of early childhood, they are learning to read and write. Each new stage of learning builds on the one before it.

Knowledge about sexuality builds much the same way. At first, your infant's understanding is entirely about their own body and senses. As they get older, they watch your behavior and continue to learn from your example. They explore on their own. They learn the words you teach them and the ideas you convey. They start to question what you say and have conversations with you.

Part II of this book is designed to give you a stage-by-stage understanding of this learning process as it relates to sexuality. It comprises five chapters:

- Chapter 6. Infants (Birth to 12 Months Old)
- Chapter 7. Toddlers (1 to 3 Years Old)
- Chapter 8. Kindergartners (4 to 6 Years Old)
- Chapter 9. In the Moment: Responding to Surprising Questions and Situations
- Chapter 10. What Comes Next?

Chapter 6
Infants
(Birth to 12 Months Old)

When parents ask us when they should start talking with their kids about sex and sexuality, we tell them that they have already started—since birth. Sexuality is about so much more than genitalia and reproduction. Infants are learning trust and attachment. They are figuring out what happens when they express their feelings and needs. They begin to learn how we value the body and its functions. We are teaching them our values about relationships and connection. They experience how we speak about and interact with their bodies, our bodies, and our partners' bodies.

Infants are deeply physically bound. They are at the very beginning stages of figuring out their bodies and how they work as mediators of the massive amounts of information in the world around them. In this year of growing and expanding senses, infants are extremely focused on the most intimate elements of sensation—with touching, listening, and seeing being the primary methods of learning about themselves and their bodies and social and cultural implications related to sexuality.

HOW INFANTS ARE LEARNING

Before we dive into the many sexuality topics infants are learning about, let's first consider four of the key *ways* infants are learning from us: feeling, listening, seeing, and intuiting.

Feeling (Physical and Emotional)

Many, although definitely not all, elements of sexuality are based in the physiological. For instance, we can detect what feels pleasant or uncomfortable in our physical body. Sexual response, including sexual pleasure, is present from before birth (Bekos & Russo, 2017). This can result in infants enjoying exploring their genitals in the same or even more focused ways than the ways they explore the rest of their bodies. Some adults are uncomfortable and react out of that discomfort when they become aware of infant masturbation. The ways that the adult reacts can set the stage for a person's understanding and judgment of their genitals and the sensations associated with them.

In addition to the sensations of touch, emotions are also physiological. Our brain detects something in our body or environment and produces a physiological reaction. As we get older, we then interpret those reactions and label them as specific feelings. This labeling process is a form of judgment on whether the physiological sensation associated with the emotions is "good" or "bad." Take, for example, the feelings associated with breastfeeding, which can include sexual stimulation. A parent's reaction to labeling that stimulation as good or bad or right or wrong is expressed from the parent to a breastfeeding infant in association with their eating.

The physiological part of sexuality is the ways that our bodies exist, the ways that our bodies feel, and how we interpret that existence and those feelings. What feels good? What feels bad? How do

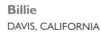

Billie
DAVIS, CALIFORNIA

Aunt and coparent to two children
Age when first became a coparent: 35

Alexander loves his penis. He's only 1, but he clearly loves touching it and playing with it. He's at that age where I guess he loves touching everything and obviously doesn't know what's what. His sister is potty training, and when she stands on her step stool to wash her hands, bare butt out before a clean diaper can be put on, he loves running up to her to try to stick his hands up her butt. It's funny at first until you realize his sister thinks it's hilarious too, and just lets him try. What a mess for everyone! It's not only his 3-year-old sister's butt he likes trying to explore, but also his own. It's so interesting watching him realize who he is in real time and explore his own body. I'm not sure what is going on up there in his head.

Diaper changes are the real hassle. Between his two hands and two legs flailing everywhere, attempting to clean his poop before he has a chance to fling it . . . it's a challenge like no other. Do most parents tackle this job with multiple people? Because it feels like this should be, at minimum, a two-person job.

The other day during a diaper change, I didn't move quickly enough, and he already had grabbed his penis and squeezed it, causing him to do that ridiculously cute laugh infants are so known for. Sticking to only the penis is manageable for me, but when he starts yanking on it and trying to use his other hand to stick up his butt, then I lose control of the situation. Sometimes giving him his own diaper wipe keeps him distracted by waving the wipe in the air. It's as if he knows his only mission, once the pants come down and the diaper is ready to be changed, is to get those tiny little hands as far up his poopy butt as possible.

At what point do you try to curb the enthusiasm and curiosity to make sure it doesn't eventually escalate toward others or in public places? I suppose when he's old enough to talk, at least he will understand what it is I'm saying. For now, it's been interesting watching him explore his own body.

those feelings arise as a result of the ways that caregivers touch and speak to an infant? When and in what context do caregivers use a certain voice or a certain touch that causes connection and closeness versus fear or trepidation?

The ways that a parent shares their own feelings and causes feelings in their child has a deep and abiding connection to the ways that infants will internalize positivity and negativity. For example, if a caregiver has a consistently negative reaction to an infant's touching their genitals—like pushing the infant's hand away—that reaction has the potential for the infant to mirror that reaction and have an internalized negative perception of their genitals without necessarily ever knowing why.

Listening

Infants, even newborns, have already been listening to the world for some time. By 18 weeks in utero, a fetus can hear sounds from inside the pregnant person's body. By 23 or 24 weeks, they can hear sounds from outside the pregnant person's body. By the time they are born, they will have an acuteness of hearing that is similar to an adult's. Their highly effective hearing and their ability to connect sounds with other stimuli allows infants as young as 6 months old to learn from our tone of voice (Zhao et al., 2019). When our infant hears us, they have an emotional response. The infant then connects those positive and negative feelings with elements of relationships and sexuality. For example, if the primary relationships around an infant are ones in which angry tones of voice are common, an infant may internalize the message that this is how intimate relationships are supposed to be.

As tones of voice are becoming clear, infants are also beginning to build their vocabularies. They are unable to control their lips, tongue, and mouth sufficiently to say many words. (Many, though, will be able to say one or two important words by the time they are 1; many will not.) However, they understand more words and, perhaps even more importantly, are learning about the process of learning words. Many infants are pointing at objects (or body parts!) as a kind of request for their parents to name the object. Parents are also pointing to objects (and body parts!) and naming them. If this process of point-and-name includes everything except the genitals, infants are learning a very clear message about what words can and cannot be said.

Talking with infants is not something that is modeled much in our culture. But there is benefit, for both parents and children, when parents are able to see their infant as someone who can hear them and learn from them and connect with them. For adults, this is often done through speech. So, even though infants can't understand all of the words and aren't able to reply back, noticeable benefits remain from having actual conversations with them beginning as early as 2 months of age (Domek et al., 2020; Shekhar et al., 2019).

Seeing

Infants start off being able to see fuzzily, without much depth, and only 8 to 12 inches away from their face—just far enough to see the face of a caregiver who is holding them. By the time they're a year old, most infants can see in many colors and with full depth perception. This exploding visual world provides a wealth of additional information. They are able to assess the positive or negative implications of facial expressions by 7 months (Ruba & Repacholi, 2020).

Most relevant to teaching about sexuality are the ways that facial expressions inform infants' assessments of positive and negative reactions on the part of their parent. Through our facial expressions, we communicate our feelings about the infant themselves, their own bodily explorations, and other elements of sexuality like anatomy, human connection, and love (Ichikawa & Yamaguchi, 2014).

Intuiting

In her book *The Highly Sensitive Child*, Elaine N. Aron wrote, "All infants are highly aware of their caregiver's feelings—their survival depends on it" (Aron, 2002, p. 56). The converging of an infant's emerging senses is what provides them with a growing intuition. Human infants have been finely tuned over millennia of evolution to understand and internalize the messages, values, and needs of their parents. And so, we, as parents, will ideally consider what we want to convey to our children about sexuality when they are still infants because we are already teaching them these things, either explicitly or implicitly.

Explicit teaching allows us to be intentional and considerate of the content in critical ways, which makes it so much better than implicit teaching! What are the messages, values, and needs that we want our children to understand? How can we live into those ideals from Day 1? Knowing these things ourselves, even at this early stage, will make it easier to impart them to our children because they are already intuiting them.

WHAT INFANTS ARE LEARNING

Although your child may currently be an infant, they are already learning the language of sexuality and the feelings around sexuality. To that end, we recommend reading through the next chapters of the book as well. This is a great time to start practicing the suggested language to use with toddlers (see Chapter 7). You can work toward saying these statements and imparting your values without worrying about the exact language. Instead, focus on the emotional messaging you're providing.

If any of the sentences we suggest in this book (including the ones from way back in Chapter 2 on self-awareness) are particularly tricky or triggering for you, practice saying a sentence aloud to your infant between birth and 6 months of age. Pay more attention to saying the words with love and care than having the exact language (Liberman et al., 2017). Your child will not connect with the actual words you are saying, but they will definitely connect with your emotional resonance. If you can become more comfortable saying anatomical body parts and connecting them with messages and values of positivity and love and safety before your infant is able to return with follow-up questions, you will have an easier time continuing this process across their lifespan. This practice also has the benefit of preparing you to just keep saying the same kinds of things to them as they age into toddlerhood, when they understand your words and begin to repeat and mimic you.

Bodies

Fetuses are learning about their bodies even before they're born. They're learning about touch, smell, taste, and sound. Among other things, this learning teaches them about physical pleasure. Fetuses have been observed touching their genitals in the uterus in rhythmic motions (Rodríguez Fernández & López Ramón y Cajal, 2016). Fetuses with penises even get erections. Infant (and toddler) penises also frequently get erect. You might notice this during diaper changes, at bath time, or first thing in the morning. This doesn't mean that they're experiencing pleasure in the same way that adults do but that the nerve endings and other tissues are working as they are designed to work.

Curiosity about their body, the sensations it brings, and an ability to explore their own genitals continues after birth. Infants often want to spend time touching their genitals during diaper changes.

What you can say:

- "You're touching your penis/vulva."
- "Oops, we don't touch poop, though! Let's wash your fingers off."
- "Oh, a little bit of spit-up. We'll just wipe that up, no problem."

Infants will also bring their curiosity to bear on the bodies of those around them. They will stick their fingers in your mouth, your ears, your eyes, everywhere! They will suck on your chin and your fingers. They will pat your cheek and your shoulder and your chest. They will grab your hair and your ears. Every way that infants try to learn about their own body, they will also try to learn about yours.

What you can say:

- "That's my ear, and I don't like it when you pull on it. Here's a toy you can pull on."
- "That's a nice, gentle way to pat me, just like I can pat you nicely and gently."

To some degree, all infant behavior is sensual because they are learning through their bodies. While some parents initially feel uncomfortable with the physical intimacy of connecting with an infant, it is actually a positive thing because of the ways that it teaches positive feelings about relationships.

Identity

Infants are learning less about who they are and more about how they are a unique, contained person who is separate from the world around them. By pushing against themselves (e.g., touching their toes, putting their fingers in their mouths) and pushing against other things (e.g., you, the bed, the floor), infants learn to distinguish the

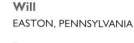

Will

EASTON, PENNSYLVANIA

Father to two children
Age when first child was born: 30

I wanted my boys to feel good about their body parts, but as a father, I had to toe the line between a positive reaction and one that might be too celebratory, and therefore, inappropriate by societal standards. This has been a recurring theme in the challenges of parenting: wanting my kids to feel good about themselves as sexual beings while also knowing that fathers who are too sex-positive come across as creepy. Dr. Ruth can talk openly about masturbation and sex toys, but this is just not as true for men.

When they were babies, I wanted to tell my boys, "Yay, you found your penis!" with the same excitement I might have if they had found their toes. But I felt I had to exercise caution about feeling too celebratory about their genitals. I have often thought about how this impacts dads. While I am making decisions about things like whether or not to show excitement over a baby finding their penis, other dads may not feel comfortable using the word "penis" at all with their kids. This is a real shame for the sexual health and well-being of everyone's children.

differences between their own body and something else in the world. Over the first year, this is a primary source of information and a key learning element.

By the end of the first year, infants have substantially different relationships with their own body, other people's bodies, and objects (and pets if you have them; Mahler et al., 2018). This relational dynamic is critical to their long-term understanding of topics like consent and boundaries (both their own and other people's).

What you can say:

- "Those are your toes! Can you imagine? All those toes, just to yourself."
- "These are my toes! You can touch them if you'd like."

In addition to grappling with the essential difference between what is ME and what is YOU, infants are already learning about relationships between other people. What kinds of relationships are possible between people? What tones of voice, facial expressions, and physical contact should be expected between two people? These are the lessons parents teach their children, intentionally or unintentionally. It's always useful to bring an intentional approach!

 What you can say:

- "I love kissing your mommy!"
- "I'm sorry I bumped into you. I'll be more careful next time" (said to your coparent/friend/family member).
- "Thank you for helping. It matters a lot to me" (said to your coparent/ friend/family member).

Emotions

Newborns express two basic emotions: attraction and withdrawal. Over the first year, infants learn all sorts of emotions, both in themselves and in others. They come to understand fear, anger, sadness, surprise, happiness, anxiety, and so much more. Even though they are, by and large, preverbal, infants can and do connect with the language of emotions: feelings (Zhao et al., 2019).

In their first 18 months of life, infants also learn about love, trust, and attachment with primary caregivers. They are learning what happens to their body when they express their feelings and needs. They are learning if the world and the people in it are essentially responsive or essentially unresponsive. This is generally called *attachment* and *attachment style* (which is different from attachment parenting). Research suggests that infants carry their basic belief systems about the responsiveness of others (or their attachment styles)—unless actively and intentionally disrupted—through childhood, adolescence, and adulthood (Lovenheim, 2018).

 What you can say:

- "I hear you crying, and I'm coming to pick you up."
- "Would you like milk? Let's see if you're hungry."
- "Do you see that red ball over there? Would you like to hold it? Here you go!"
- "I love you."

Boundaries

Boundaries can be hard to figure out with infants. Newborns are broadly unaware of where their body stops and starts, but they can still cause hurt and injury to those around them.

One of Karen's good friends had her cornea sliced by her newborn's fingernail as the child's hands were flailing about one day. (It healed, no long-term damage!) There is little that could have been done to prevent this accident. But by the time a baby turns 1 and is solidly on their way to being a toddler, they should have substantial control over their large body movements and know how to keep their hands away from someone's eyeball. On the other hand, infants need an immense amount of physical closeness to develop the kinds of trust and connection that lead to long-term healthy approaches to relationships. Finding a balance of teaching infants about appropriate boundaries while remaining close to them during a period of immense growth and preverbal communication is a tricky thing.

Let's take breastfeeding as an example. Breastfeeding can be painful because of the way an infant is approaching it, and yet it is still necessary for a breastfeeding infant to participate in the process. While some people enjoy breastfeeding their infants, others find the sensation annoying or even painful. If this is the case for you, trust that your body should not be in pain. Seek out a breastfeeding consultant to help check your child's latch and other elements of the breastfeeding relationship, and make corrections as possible. *Arranging an environment that sets up an infant to not breach a boundary is a first and critical step.*

When your infant starts teething, they are more likely to squeeze things between their gums because it feels good to them. You can gently and immediately unlatch and stop them from breastfeeding. Tell them that they have hurt you and then let them return to breastfeeding. If they bite you again, unlatch and hold them slightly farther away from your body for a slightly longer time and tell them again that they have hurt you. Infants can learn when it is okay to bite down on something and when it is not. *Responding with kindness and firmness when an infant hurts you or someone else begins to teach them what is approved touch and what is not. Continue to be kind and firm in these steps, even if your child cries and is upset.*

These early lessons on consent and boundaries, particularly when they're taught with love and gentleness, lead directly into conversations with toddlers, young children, older children, and eventually teenagers about how to listen to the needs of others and how to expect that others will listen to our needs.

 What you can say:

- "You're biting me, and that hurts. Let's get you something that you can bite all you want."
- "Your fingernail scratched me! Let's go cut them so they won't hurt you or me or anyone else."
- "When you pull my hair, it hurts, and it's important not to hurt people, so let's unwind your finger, and then you can hold my finger."

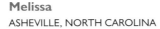

Melissa

ASHEVILLE, NORTH CAROLINA

Mother to two children
Age when first child was born: 29

Babies are so beautifully, vociferously clear about their boundaries! I've been trying to help River learn to watch for nonverbal cues about consent (or lack thereof) in a variety of situations, and it's so helpful for him to see how Hazel clearly expresses her feelings about what's happening to her body, even though she's still a preverbal baby! If she doesn't like something (like when he puts something on her head or tries to pick her up), she just cries. And then he understands, "Oh, she doesn't like that!" His care for his sister means that he's more willing to adapt to what she needs. Even if he has a hard time stopping a certain behavior when we ask him to, he listens to Hazel's clear, embodied "No!" right away.

Hazel is also now pushing people's hands away and showing other signals that she doesn't like something before starting to cry, which is helpful for him to see. We're trying to help him notice the signs that she's overwhelmed or doesn't like a certain kind of game or touch before she starts to cry, and he's getting better at it. (And then, we're also extrapolating to practice those observations in other scenarios, with older kids and with us, since he's a very tactile, exuberant kid.)

I wonder what the world would be like if we kept our early clarity about our bodily boundaries? If it stayed okay for us to express them clearly, and if others honored that, rather than telling kids they "have to" hug someone because it's expected or "polite"? Babies don't care if they "hurt someone's feelings" by crying to say, "No, I don't like that!" When and why do we lose that capacity?

And yet, there's also some uncertainty about how to navigate Hazel's cries when it's not an optional touch, like when she really needs a diaper change! We're doing our best to be respectful about it, to tell her what needs to happen and why, and to empathize with her feelings about it. That's leading to good conversations with River too, about what types of touch for health and safety are necessary versus what's negotiable. So many nuances! And, it's harder to have these conversations when I didn't have them as a kid myself; changing the narrative and the daily practice is hard work!

We know that parenting an infant is an intense experience. A new baby is exciting, and infants are precious and delightful! And they are also 24/7 intensity. As parents we are often sleep deprived and just trying to figure out what the baby needs at any given moment while trying to juggle our own needs and sometimes the needs of other little (and big!) people in our family. The more compassion (positivity/forgiveness) we can have for ourselves in this process, the more we can ask others for support and meet our own needs, and the more we will be able to convey those positive feelings to our baby and have the capacity to think about things like the material in this book.

SUMMARY

Infants are already learning so many things from their parents—from language to emotion to connection. When parents bring awareness and intentionality to their interactions around physical response, pleasure, connection, language, and other sexuality adjacent topics, they set up a household culture that will sustain dialogue and education and safety throughout the infant's lifespan.

RESOURCES FOR PARENTS

Online

- American Academy of Pediatrics parenting website: https://healthychildren.org/English/Pages/default.aspx

Book

- *Developing Self and Self-Concepts in Early Childhood Education and Beyond* by Bridie Raban (Emerald Publishing)

Chapter 7
Toddlers
(1 to 3 Years Old)

The great majority of people we talk with become interested in the topics covered in this book after their child is no longer an infant. If you are learning about childhood sexuality while your child is a toddler, that's fantastic. Don't worry or feel guilty that you didn't read about it earlier. Toddlerhood is a brilliant time to start teaching your child about sexuality as they tip into being verbal.

Toddlers are excellent sex ed students. They are wired for curiosity and learning. Toddler curiosity can be a big help as we do our job of teaching them about healthy sexuality. They want to know the names of things and how things are categorized. They have a pureness of wonder that allows them to soak up information without the layers of social stigma. In addition to being curious, toddlerhood is a time when we see a massive shift in verbal development as children become able to name things and then string together sentences. Although our attitudes and behaviors remain key to effectively teaching our own kiddo, we can now start to give them a lot more verbal information too.

Another reason that toddlers make great sex ed students is that they aren't self-conscious yet. They cannot see themselves from someone else's point of view. They don't get embarrassed (Buss et al., 1979). Sometimes this can be awkward for us caregivers. One parent told Laura about a time when they were grocery shopping, and their child loudly pronounced, "My penis is hard, and it feels funny!" While instances such as this may make us red in the face, we can use the unashamed toddler phase to our advantage. Think back to the exercise you did naming reproductive anatomy out loud in Chapter 2. If you felt a bit squeamish with any of those terms (or maybe all of them!), remember that your child will have none of those awkward or uncomfortable feelings as you teach them about sexuality. They're starting with a blank slate in this regard. If you can regulate your own discomfort around sexual topics beforehand, your child can learn about sexuality without associated shame.

Speaking of embarrassing or shocking moments, one goal of this chapter is to help you know what kinds of behavior are typical for toddlers. We continue to give you examples of real-life situations and stories about kids and sexuality. One of our hopes is that you will come to recognize normal toddler behavior so you can feel more relaxed when it happens with your child and more confident in how you respond. Chapter 5 has information to help you know when you should investigate more to make sure that your child hasn't been exposed to inappropriate behavior or abuse. Just as important, we want you to know that you are not alone. Talk with the parents of toddlers and preschoolers about the things kids do that are related to bodies and sexuality, and, like us, you'll get to hear an amazing array of stories. We encourage you to try it.

What follows is a discussion of the sexuality topics you can teach your child during toddlerhood as well as practical ways you can teach them. There are many opportunities in daily life to teach little kids about sexuality. In this chapter, we help you to recognize the teachable moments that arise spontaneously and offer you ideas for how to proactively create teachable moments for your toddler.

HOW TODDLERS ARE LEARNING

Before we dive into the many sexuality topics toddlers are learning about, let's first consider the three key *ways* toddlers learn from us about sexuality: touching, observing and imitating (play), and listening and asking.

Touching

One of the primary means by which toddlers are learning about sexuality is through touch. Just like infants, toddlers experience love and nurturing through physical care and affection. Touch and physical comfort play a central role in forming and maintaining attachments, helping toddlers regulate their emotions, and meeting their other needs for touch. Touch also provides a lot of information as kids investigate their world. As a result, they try to touch and feel everything they can with their hands and mouth. Here are typical sexual behaviors we see in toddlers that involve touch:

- touching their own genitals or nipples in private or public
- masturbating
- touching the bodies of caregivers, including grasping breasts or genitals
- touching, grasping at, or looking at genitals or breasts of other adults
- touching the bodies of other children during play, including genitals

Observing and Imitating (Play)

Kids in this age group are astute observers. This is one reason why modeling healthy behavior and attitudes is key to teaching healthy sexuality. During this stage, children watch adults closely and then mimic the behavior they see (Newton et al., 2016). They imitate cooking, breastfeeding, working on a computer, pregnancy, and just about anything else that interests them.

To illustrate, here is a story about a time when Laura was baby-sitting the 3-year-old of a close friend. Let's call the toddler "Noa." It was a hot day, and Noa was wearing only her underwear. At some point, Laura noticed Noa had a big bulge in her underpants. She took a minute to consider what this might be. It didn't smell or look like poop. In her most nonchalant voice, Laura asked, "Oh, hey, what's in your underpants?" Noa got a little shy and took a washcloth out of her underwear. Laura just said, "Oh, okay." Laura didn't inquire any further but planned to talk with Noa's mother about what had happened. It wasn't until a couple of hours later that she realized what her little friend was doing: Noa had been imitating using cloth menstrual pads, just like her mother.

Listening and Asking

Another way toddlers learn is through what they hear. They begin to understand what we say before they begin to talk, and they tend to hear much more than we think they do. They hear, for instance, what we say about bodies, bodily functions, love, and relationships. They also pick up on our tone of voice. In addition, toddlers begin to ask a wonderful array of direct questions. This is a list of some real questions that toddlers have asked (example answers to these questions are provided in Chapter 9):

- Is that a man or a woman?
- How did the baby get in there?
- How did the baby come out?
- What is that? (Asked while pointing to any array of objects, including tampons, vibrators, or anything else they find)

- Why can't I come into the bathroom?
- Where's your penis?
- Why do you have hair *there*?
- Why is your butt so jiggly?

Keep in mind that toddler questions aren't inherently offensive because we know it's a toddler's job to be curious and to try to understand the world. Even so, these kinds of questions (or their statements) can be embarrassing when others overhear them or when they might offend someone. They can also be uncomfortable

Judith

AMSTERDAM, THE NETHERLANDS

Mother to two children
Age when first child was born: 22

Last week, Siem was walking around the house in his flannel pajamas, carrying his stuffed toy in one hand and a sandwich in the other. He opened the door to our bedroom and saw Daan getting dressed. I think it must have been the first time he had seen Daan naked and actually realized it.

Siem walked back to the living room where I was, looked at me with absolute amazement in his eyes, and said, "Daddy has a willie! Siemie has willie too." I could see his eyes changing emotion as a thought came to him. He looked at me and asked, "Mommy willie too?" When I said that I didn't have one because mommies don't have willies, his eyes got even bigger with amazement than before.

The next time I got dressed, he came in to check! Now, his new game is asking everyone who comes to our house if they have a willie, including the mailman and grandma. I am glad that he chose our "fun" granny to ask. If he would have asked our other granny, she might have choked on her tea!

when we don't know how to respond and how much information to provide. In this chapter as well as in Chapter 9, we help you prepare for such moments.

WHAT TODDLERS ARE LEARNING

Now that we have considered some of the ways toddlers are learning, let's jump into the things they are learning *about*. Many parents are anxious to know which topics are okay to discuss with their kids. In this section, we provide details about the sexuality topics that are particularly beneficial to help your child start to learn while they are toddlers—whether or not your child asks about them. Your child may ask you about other topics. *Any topic that comes up in your toddler's life is fair game for discussion.* The key is to regulate yourself and adjust the depth and complexity of your responses to your child's stage of comprehension. Here, we help you to do that by supplying example language and dialogues and offering other tools for teaching.

Next, we describe ways you can incorporate learning about sexual health into daily life. Remember that these ideas are meant to be relayed in many little, separate conversations that happen throughout your child's life. As children get older, you can have more in-depth conversations about more complicated topics. Even then, make chats about sexual health part of an ongoing dialogue rather than one or even a few big talks.

As you teach these ideas, you'll notice that young children need repetition. Your child will benefit if you repeat many times over the years the knowledge you are teaching them about sexual health.

Bodies

Bodies are a big part of what composes our understanding of sexuality. How we think and feel about the physical body and the bodies of others, what physical boundaries we set, what we do with our body, and how we talk about bodies are all important parts of sexual health. Moreover, toddlers' lives are grounded in physical experiences. At this stage, teaching kids about bodies is a central theme when communicating about healthy sexuality.

How We Value the Body, Diversity, and Bodily Functions

As we've discussed earlier about infants, we are still teaching our toddler how we value the body, including body parts and bodily functions. We want to help our child grow into an adult who feels proud of their body for its uniqueness and strengths. We want to teach them to feel ownership over what happens with their body and responsibility for its care. To develop these attitudes, we can show them that we have positive feelings about their body and ours. We can show them that all parts of the body—from head to toe—have important functions. One of the ways we demonstrate our values about the body is through the names and attention we give to the different parts of the body, which we discuss shortly.

Kids learn how we think and feel about bodies by how we talk about them. If we are in the habit of criticizing our own body in front of our child or commenting about other people's bodies (positively or negatively), we are also teaching them to be critical of their own body and other people's bodies. Instead, we can help our child to appreciate physical diversity. While there are many similarities among human bodies, every body is also unique. No two bodies look or work exactly the same. Appreciating this uniqueness can help your child understand that other kids and adults will not be like them or their family. Teaching about physical variation is one way to teach about the beauty of diversity and how much we appreciate individual uniqueness.

In later years, kids will begin to compare themselves with others. Knowing that all bodies are different can help your child to feel good about themselves when they aren't the same as their peers. At the same time, it will help children appreciate differences in others' bodies, including appearances, abilities, and disabilities.

 What you can say:

- "All bodies are unique. There are no two bodies that are exactly the same, even in twins. Isn't that amazing?"
- "You are the only person exactly like YOU. I like it that we aren't all the same. It's fun to see different bodies in the world."
- "Look how capable you are!"
- "Is your tummy growling? It's so cool that our bodies tell us when we need something like that. How does your body tell you when it's tired?"

Another way we convey our feelings about the body is how we react to and discuss bodily functions like burping, farting, peeing, and pooping. All these bodily functions are normal, and, at first, they are all appropriate to do in public—babies do all these things and more regardless of who is there with them. As kids get older, we help them to understand what behaviors are appropriate in which contexts.

A big milestone for toddlers that involves bodily functions is learning to use the toilet. However we choose to help our child transition out of diapers and onto the pot, we also have a choice about the attitudes we take toward things like peeing and pooping. In short, try to keep it positive. Whether our child is getting a diaper change or is sitting on the toilet, we can celebrate that their body is working properly to flush out the stuff it doesn't need. An extra stinky poop can be a laughable moment rather than an eye-rolling "Eww." (It's okay to get out the air freshener.)

When they start learning to use the toilet, and even before, many kids are fascinated by peeing and pooping. Kids are often intrigued by excrement. "What does my poop look like today?"

might be a familiar question in your home too. One 3-year-old Laura knew would sit on the toilet and ask Laura to read her a four-page section of a book that illustrated where pee and poop come from. The toddler wanted these pages to be read over and over and over again. This kind of behavior and interest in elimination are typical. Toddlers are intrigued by the changing color and smell of urine or about the different ways one can get it into the toilet. It is all perfectly normal.

 What you can say:

- "Thanks for telling me you need to pee."
- "You are peeing a lot today. That means you are drinking enough and staying hydrated."
- "I know! That was a stinky one! Your body must be doing a good job getting rid of all the stuff it doesn't need."

GENITALS: NAMING AND EXPLORING

We often see young kids learning about minute details of their anatomy, such as their eyelashes, eyebrows, eyelids, teeth, tongue, and gums. They learn where their stomach and heart are inside their body. These are really fun things to teach kids about, and kids are fascinated by how the body works. But, there is often something missing when we teach them all those cool things about the body: We skip over genitals. When caregivers do provide names for genitals, we sometimes use slang terms to generally describe an entire area. Rather than teach kids specific terms, such as *penis* and *scrotum*, we might say they have a "wee-wee." Instead of telling kids, "That is a *vulva* and *vagina*," we might say they are "lady bits." Or, instead of using the term *anus*, we might call the whole backside the "bum."

Using these casual terms can help *us* feel more comfortable, but what messages are we sending to our kids when we make the entire genital region a gray area with a funny name? Combined with the fact that genitalia are often covered up for sanitation purposes or privacy, using slang terms can send a message to children that there is something secret or forbidden about them. Moreover, it teaches kids that we don't talk openly about them. On the other hand, using accurate anatomical terms sends the message that genitals are just as important and wonderful as the rest of the body. It says we can talk directly and openly about them without shame or discomfort. Importantly, teaching kids the proper terms for genitals and that genitals are an open topic of conversation in your family can also help protect them from child sexual abuse or help your child tell you if abuse has occurred.

Children are not inherently embarrassed about genitalia or bodily functions, but that's not always true for adults. Both of us are sexual health educators, and there have still been times when we have talked with our children about sexual topics and felt a little weird or didn't know exactly what to say in the moment. You can get more comfortable by using anatomical terms on your own, with other parents who are learning the same thing, or even as you use the terms with your child.

The anatomical terms we can start using with infants and toddlers are *anus, clitoris, penis, scrotum, testes, urethra, uterus, vagina,* and *vulva.* If you aren't familiar with these terms, see the diagrams and descriptions of them in Chapter 3.

Even though genitals are often covered up by clothing, we have many opportunities to teach kids about them. When your child is in the bathtub, you can play a naming game. Take turns pointing to a body part for the other person to identify. Name genitals that are clearly in view just like you would any other body part (e.g., vulva, penis).

In addition to their own anatomy, teach children about other kinds of genitals. A useful way to teach these terms is through anatomically correct dolls and toys. A few brands of dolls are anatomically correct, which means they have genitalia. If you only get one doll, get a doll that has different genitals from your child. That will give you and your child the chance to discuss different bodies. Doll brands we recommend and other anatomically correct toys are listed in our Resources for Kids section at the end of this chapter.

Books are another fantastic resource, and we have listed several toddler-appropriate books in the Resources for Kids section too. Keep in mind that kids at this stage haven't started thinking abstractly yet. In other words, they understand what they can see. Conversely, they won't easily understand a drawing of something inside the body. Drawings in younger toddlers books are usually simple and focus on external anatomy. From ages 3 to 5 years old, children begin to understand diagrams that represent things they cannot actually see, like internal anatomy. When they are ready, books with internal anatomy are important because they give kids anatomical terms for when they learn how babies are made.

 What you can say:

- "Your pee comes out of the urethra."
- "It looks like your vulva is a little red. Does it feel sore?"
- "Your penis has a foreskin, that bit right there."
- "Let's get your anus clean now that you're finished pooping."

Along with learning the correct names for genitals, young kids also learn that genitals are an area of the body that are particularly sensitive and may feel good to touch. Many kids explore how their genitals feel. Even if they aren't playing with their genitals per se, just covering genitals with one's hands is a soothing feeling for many people. Other children find that rubbing their nipples is a soothing feeling that helps to reduce stress. Toddlers haven't learned about social boundaries yet, including the difference between what we consider public and private. You may find your child playing with their genitals or masturbating out in the open. This is normal. At times

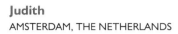

Judith
AMSTERDAM, THE NETHERLANDS

Mother to two children
Age when first child was born: 22

I was changing Siem's diaper in his room today, and we were playing a game in which I named body parts, and he pointed them out. It's a pretty routine game for us by now. He pointed to his eyes, ears, nose, and legs and then pointed to mine. Then he pointed at his navel and asked, "Penis?" I was a bit unsure about what to do. He never asked about that before. My mind was racing through the nonexistent lessons about our private parts that I had as a kid and about how unsure it still makes me. Then I decided to just go with it, and I pointed out his penis. Of course, he pointed out my crotch next, asking, "Penis?" again, and I told him women don't have a penis. It was my breasts' turn after that. I gave him the name for those too. Now they are just another part of our game routine.

I still feel a little bit weird about it, but talking about it becomes easier every time. Yesterday, we were sitting in our garden, and he was sitting on my lap. I was talking to Daan, and Siem grabbed the top of my shirt, pulled it open, looked inside, and yelled, "Cheeks! Mommy's got cheeks!" Daan almost peed his pants laughing. I think we must subtly teach Siem about what is appropriate and what is not at some point.

like this, we want to acknowledge that self-touch is pleasurable, that many people like it, *and* that it's private.

Toddlerhood is a good time to bring up the topics of pleasure and soothing in general as well. While they are certainly becoming more verbal and cognitive, toddlers are still rooted in their physical body. They explore what feels good and continue to do those things that they like. Help your toddler identify and express their preferences for what feels good to them. Do they like back scratches, or do those tickle? Do they enjoy the cold or prefer cozy warmth? Do they like cuddles and kisses or need more space? Maybe they like the feel of particular fabrics on their skin.

This is an area of sexuality that requires some introspection and processing for many adults if we are going to pass on healthy attitudes to our child. Adults in the United States are often uncomfortable talking about pleasure, especially sexual pleasure. When it comes to young kids, many of us don't talk about pleasure because we don't want to oversexualize our child. We are afraid that talking to kids about reproduction and especially about pleasure is inappropriate and could be damaging. To be clear, we don't want to explicitly detail adult sexual behaviors, but we can acknowledge a child's own experience in ways that are devoid of shame. One additional aspect of this topic to consider is the gender difference in attitudes about pleasure. While pleasure-seeking is considered normal and often encouraged in boys, it is often ignored or discouraged when it comes to girls. This is a disparity we can help to change.

 What you can say:

- "Hey, kiddo. It's totally fine if you want to touch your penis/vulva. Many people enjoy doing that with their body because it feels good, but it's a private thing, so will you do it in the bedroom?"
- "Playing with your genitals is something we do in private."

PUBERTY: HOW KID BODIES BECOME ADULT BODIES

As we've said earlier, any topic that your child brings up is fair game for discussion, and you can address it with truthful, age-appropriate information. Your toddler will, of course, not sit you down for a serious one-to-one conversion and ask you about puberty. However, there are many opportunities for teaching about it. As toddlers explore their world, they notice differences between themselves and the adults around them. Some adults have breasts or hair in places that kids don't (like whiskers on the face or hair on the armpits or genitals). When kids notice these differences between kids and adults, we have a great chance to tell them that there's a particular time when a kid's body changes into an adult one: puberty. We don't need to go into all the details, but we can tell them what it is called and talk about some of the changes that occur during puberty.

Many people have grown up not feeling particularly well prepared for the jumble of hormonal roller coasters called puberty. Consider how you learned about puberty. Did you feel well prepared? Now consider what your experience would have been if, like the other topics in this book, puberty was an open topic of conversation *from the beginning*? What would it look like if your toddler or kindergartner knew what puberty is and learned more and more details about it as they got older? Kids can start a normal pubertal process as early as 8 years old. Even if they aren't going through it themselves at age 8, some of your child's classmates may be. When children are 7 years old, we can start teaching them more comprehensively about puberty. We know that sounds really young, but don't put it off! If your child learns about puberty from the beginning, it will already be a familiar concept.

 What you can say:

- "I have hair on my vulva because I'm a grown-up. Right now, you're a kid, so you don't have that. When you're older, your body will change into an adult body. You will get hair around your genitals and in your armpits too."
- "The time when our bodies change from being a kid body to an adult body is called puberty. The body changes a lot during puberty."
- "That's called deodorant. People put it under their arms, in their armpits, to help them not smell or sweat so much. That's something that happens when you go through puberty; you'll get hair under your armpits and also sweat and smell more."
- "People with a uterus start to get their period after they go through puberty and get an adult body."

Boundaries: Body Safety and Consent

If you have not yet read Chapter 5 about child sexual abuse, we encourage you to do so. Toddlerhood is a very important time to focus on teaching about body safety and consent. At this stage, teaching about boundaries requires a consistent effort because toddlers don't have a good internal sense of which touch is appropriate and which is not. This is a time when you will have ongoing opportunities to remind your child over and over about ideas that can help to keep them safer. We want children to know that their body is their own and they get to have agency over it, especially when it comes to genitals.

 What you can say (in addition to our suggestions in Chapter 5):

- "Genitals are private."
- "Your genitals are special, and no one except you should touch them. Sometimes a doctor might need to help you with your genitals if you're not feeling well, but it should always be when I am there with you."
- "There are still some things I need to help you with, like wiping poops, but, otherwise, you get to decide how people touch your body."
- "You can come to me or [name another trusted adult] any time you have a question or feel uncomfortable. I won't be mad at you."
- "You don't want to give kisses? Okay, would you like to do fist bumps, high fives, or blow kisses?"
- "Sarah, let's ask Letisha if she would like to hug bye-bye."
- "It looks like your friend doesn't want hugs right now. Why don't we ask if they would like us to blow them a kiss instead?"
- To an adult: "I know it's different from what you are used to. A lot of research has now been done on how to teach kids about safety, and it's recommended that kids get to choose how and when to be affectionate—even with family."

One way we can start to show toddlers that their genitals are only for them to touch (except in very particular circumstances) is at bath time. We find that kids often need help rinsing shampoo out of their hair, but, otherwise, toddlers are capable of cleaning their own body, especially their genitals. Letting a child wash their own genitals is a concrete way of showing them that their genitals are off-limits except in very specific circumstances. In the end, a soak in the tub works well to get them clean. If you feel that their anus should be cleaned with mild soap, allowing your child to clean their own anus teaches them that they have control over what happens with their genitals.

 What you can say:

- "You're old enough now that you can wash yourself if you would like to. Do you want to use the soap on your anus? Or would you prefer that I help you?"
- "Your genitals are only for you to touch. Sometimes a grown-up might need to help you, like with a messy poop, but that should only be [use specific names]."

Teaching about boundaries and body safety also requires teaching about privacy. Which parts of our bodies are private? What behaviors are appropriate in different contexts? Every family has different levels of comfort when it comes to privacy and nudity. Whatever those boundaries are for your family, teaching children the concept of privacy is important. You can start by modeling. Talk about needing privacy for yourself, even if that's a couple minutes of time alone in the bathroom. Toddlers don't typically want privacy for themselves (we see this more in the kindergarten years), but it's good for them to understand the concept. If your family is particularly open, this may be easier to do when nonfamily members are in the home. You can explain, for example, that you are closing the bathroom door for privacy when guests are in the house.

Toddlers can learn the difference between acceptable behavior inside the privacy of their home compared with what behaviors are appropriate out in public. What you and your family find appropriate depends on your comfort level, what you have decided you want your child to learn, and the norms of the culture in which you live. As a parent, it's fine to be naked in front of your child, regardless of your anatomy or your child's. If parents of more than one sex are living in the household, it's helpful for kids to see all kinds of bodies. If you aren't comfortable with this, then don't do it. You should, however, make sure your child sees nonsexualized naked bodies. Fact-based kids' books or games about anatomy are a good resource for this (see the suggestions in the Resources for Kids section at the end of this chapter).

When naked or bathing around your child, they may touch your body or ask questions. If they are touching your genitals, use the situation as an opportunity to teach boundaries. You can gently remove their hand and remind them that your genitals are only for you. You will very likely have to repeat this routine, just like you would for any other boundaries you set with toddlers. Likewise, kids may also be curious about the genitalia of friends or siblings. They may show each other their genitals and even include genitals in games, such as playing doctor. This is normal. It is our job to teach them about boundaries without shaming them for displaying normal behavior.

With regard to nudity and genitalia specifically, we want to teach kids that genitals are special without instilling shame about them. Whether or not you prefer that your child covers their genitals at home and in public, it is important to let them know that their genitals are theirs and for no one else to touch unless they need help from you. Kids often enjoy being naked. Toddlers typically won't mind at all being naked in front of other people. Depending on their toilet habits, and your tolerance for accidents, you can allow your child to be naked around your home, in the yard, or in other places outdoors. This gives them the opportunity to explore their body, and that's a good thing. If you don't want them running around naked and they only check out their genitals during baths and diaper changes, that's fine too.

Many parents ask when they should stop being naked in front of their child, stop bathing with their child, or stop siblings from bathing together. As a rule of thumb, *as soon as anyone in the situation (adult or child) indicates that they are uncomfortable for any reason, that's the time to stop.*

What you can say:

- "That's my penis/vulva. I know it's so interesting, but my genitals are for me."
- "That part of the body belongs to me only."
- "I know that you are really curious about bodies, and that's super cool, but people's genitals are only for them. Let's go look at a book about bodies instead."

Billie
DAVIS, CALIFORNIA

Aunt and coparent to two children
Age when first became a coparent: 35

Mia loves going up to me or her mom to immediately put her hands up our shirts and grab our boobs to remind us that she's thirsty. Jen is still breastfeeding Alexander, so while Mia is not actively breastfeeding, she still remembers it's something Jen used to do with her. She asks me if she can have some of my milk, and I have to remind her that I don't have any breast milk, that not every woman with breasts has milk, and that it's not appropriate to go to women other than mommy to ask about their breast milk.

Yesterday, the kids were both jumping on the bed, and she hopped on me, asking to see my boobs, but before I could answer, she lifted my shirt and tried squeezing them. It was innocent, of course, but it got me thinking about how this could be a valuable lesson to introduce the idea about consent. Even at 3, she has a really good sense of herself and lets us know when she wants to be hugged or kissed, so it's not a totally foreign concept.

"Sweetie," I said. "I don't want to show you my boobs right now." And in classic toddler form, she ignored what I said and kept trying. It seemed like a game at first; Alexander was sitting next to me, laughing at her attempts. "Baby, no, I don't want you to put your hands up my shirt." She got mad: "NO. But I want to." I lifted her off of me and placed her next to her brother. "But, sweetie, I said NO. What do we do when somebody says no?" She made an overly quizzical expression and with conviction said, "Can I see your boobies and milk, PLEASE?" Wow. I don't know why I wasn't expecting that response. Walked right into that, didn't I?

"Well," I laughed, "No, but thank you for saying please." Hmm, this was harder than I realized. I continued, "If someone STILL SAYS NO, what should we do?" She crossed her arms and didn't say anything. She just looked so angry and confused: "FINE. I don't want to see them anymore." She clearly was backpedaling and tried to distract herself by playing with her brother.

"Baby," I said. "You know how you don't like to hug some people sometimes? And you tell them no, thank you?" She nodded. "Well, this is like that. It's called consent. I know this word doesn't mean anything to you right now," I laughed. "But it means . . . like . . . someone allows you to do something. If someone tells you no, you need to respect their wishes. When you listen, that's consent. Does that make sense?" She nodded, "Even if I say pretty please?" I nodded with a smile. "Yes, dear, even if you say pretty please." She likes to elongate her words sarcastically, and that's usually how I know I've gotten through to her. "Alllllll riiiiiight. I get it." We'll see how long that lasts, but it was a good first start!

Babies

Toddlerhood is a natural time to teach about how babies are made. Between the ages of 1 and 3 is a time when many children learn that a younger sibling will be joining the family. If your toddler isn't going to become a big sibling, chances are that some of their friends will have a pregnant parent. This is a time when kids often ask questions like, "How did the baby get in there?" Or, "How does it get out?" Although it's a natural time to discuss these topics, many parents feel uncomfortable, not wanting to give too much information too early. You *can* address these touchy topics in honest, age-appropriate ways.

REPRODUCTION: CONCEPTION, PREGNANCY, AND BIRTH

By 3 years old, toddlers are capable of understanding the basics of menstruation, conception, pregnancy, birth, and baby care. You may be thinking, "Wait. What? I'm going to teach my toddler about reproduction?!" The idea may seem strange, but we are here to help you. Your first conversations about reproduction are going to be very short and simple. Remember that by starting these small conversations early, we parents get to practice discussing important topics so that we're ready for the bigger conversations later on. In addition, we make it clear from the beginning that we are their go-to source of information about these kinds of important topics.

When toddlers are first learning about reproduction, we can teach them many things. Some examples of how to talk with a toddler about conception, pregnancy, and birth follow shortly. If a child is already familiar with the correct terminology for reproductive anatomy, it makes these conversations a bit easier. These discussion ideas are meant to be used little by little, over time. We start with small and simple bits of information. Then we repeat what we want them to

Florence

AMSTERDAM, THE NETHERLANDS

Mother to two children
Age when first child was born: 40

Just before she turned 4, my daughter was asking a lot of questions about marriage, partnership, and who lives with whom. One evening at a family dinner with my parents, she declared, "When I grow up, I want to marry Mommy and Daddy and live with them forever." We all thought this was super cute until she went on saying, "And I also think I will want to have children. So then Daddy will be the sperm." My parents are not so open about these things, so you can imagine the awkward silence that ensued. I tried to reply in a positive way (knowing that she'll understand when she's older why that's not a going to happen), but all that came out was, "Yay! Then we can all live together forever!"

know and add more details over time. You know your child best, and you can gauge how much information to give at one time and when it is a good time to add more.

What you can say:

- "To make a baby, there needs to be an egg from one person and sperm from another person. Then the baby grows inside a part of the body called the uterus."
- "An egg is so small that we can barely see it, and sperm are so small that we can only see them if we have a special tool called a microscope. When an egg and sperm get together, they can grow bigger and bigger until a baby is ready to be born."
- "When an egg and sperm first come together, they don't look like a baby. Here are some pictures of what a baby looks like as it grows in the uterus."

163

- "People with a vulva and vagina usually have a uterus. They also usually have breasts to feed the baby milk after it is born."
- "Before a baby is born, we sometimes call it a fetus."
- "After many, many months of waiting, the baby lets the uterus know that it is ready to come out. Then the uterus pushes the baby out through the vagina."
- "The vagina is like a stretchy tube. The opening to the vagina is different from the urethra (where the pee comes out) or anus (where the poop comes out), but it's in the same area."
- "The entrance to the vagina is in between the urethra (in the front) and the anus (in the back)."
- "When you were born . . ." (Many children love to hear their birth story!)

MENSTRUATION

Menstruation is another topic related to conception. Although menstruation is not a subject that is especially important for toddlers, if someone in the household is menstruating regularly, that provides learning opportunities. Why not take advantage of them? In addition, it's good to be prepared in case your child asks you about menstrual pads, tampons, or other things associated with menstruation.

 What you can say:

- "This is my pad/tampon/cup. I use it to catch the blood that comes from my uterus. That happens every once in a while, and it's normal. I'm not hurt in any way."
- "Each month, blood builds up around the walls of the uterus to make a nice little place for a baby to grow. If no baby is growing in my uterus, then my body flushes out the blood, and it comes out of my vagina. Then new, fresh blood builds up in the uterus again."
- "The body lines the uterus with blood in case a person becomes pregnant. If they do get pregnant, the baby will grow in the uterus, and the blood will stay there. If the person doesn't become pregnant, the blood comes out through the vagina."

Families

As you know very well, babies and kids need a lot of care, and they get that care from a family. But what makes a family, exactly? Is everyone in a family biologically related? Does everyone in a family have to live together? How many moms or dads are there in a family? Can kids live with other people besides a parent?

Sometimes we go about our interactions with other families without ever explicitly discussing how families can be different. When you take the time to point out various family structures, your child learns about diversity. They learn that other kids live in circumstances different from theirs. A fun way to talk about different kinds of families is through stories and books like the ones we have recommended at the end of the chapter. If you have examples of different family structures from your own social sphere, pointing those out can also be helpful.

 What you can say:

- "Families can look a lot of different ways. Some kids live with only one parent; other kids live with two moms or two dads."
- "Some kids have parents in different houses."
- "Some kids live with grandparents or other relatives."
- "An adoption is when someone (or several people) become parents for a child who doesn't have parents who can care for them."

Gender Identity, Expression, and Roles

In Chapter 4, we discussed some important ideas and terminology around gender. Increasingly, parents are becoming aware of the expectations we place on children based on gender and are working toward a less gendered (or in some cases nongendered) way of parenting. In addition, we are becoming continuously more aware of children whose gender identity is different from the sex they were assigned at birth. In all, children and adults are now finding more freedom to express their gender in nontraditional ways.

When kids are in the early part of toddlerhood, they don't yet understand our cultural ideas around gender. They have to be taught how to use pronouns, for example, and they often use incorrect pronouns at first. Toddlers are also not yet particularly concerned with their own gender. A 2-year-old will imitate an adult regardless of the adult's gender, and they are not concerned with whether a toy is supposed to be for boys or girls. In these early years, they are often happy to wear any clothing they are given, regardless of color or style. As toddlers get older, usually around the age of 3, they may become more interested in gender identity and expression. This phenomenon intensifies the more they are around similar-age peers (Halim et al., 2018).

How a parent approaches teaching their child about gender is a very personal decision. What we find most important is that parents explicitly discuss the fact that a person's gender identity or gender expression does not tell us what their genitals look like. It's also helpful to discuss that we can't always assume a person's gender.

In our Resources for Kids section, we include books to read to your child that encourage discussion about gender identity. We have also included resources to help you learn more about different ways of approaching gender with your child.

 What you can say:

- "When babies are born, parents usually look at their genitals and then decide if the baby is a boy or a girl. If the baby has a vulva and vagina, they say it's a girl. If the baby has a penis and scrotum, they say it's a boy. But not all people feel like they are a boy or girl just because their parents said so."
- "People like to dress in different ways, no matter if they are a boy or a girl."
- "Some people don't want to say if they are a girl or a boy."
- "We don't know what someone's body is like under their clothes. That's really their own business."

Feelings

Understanding and processing our emotions is key to personal health and healthy relationships. If you've parented a toddler, you know they have big feelings! On top of that, toddlers can evoke big feelings in *us*. Those strong emotions can be opportunities to help us teach toddlers about feelings (Poulin-Dubois et al., 2018). For toddlers, we can start by mirroring and labeling feelings that a child might be experiencing at a given moment. When we mirror a child's feelings by using similar facial expressions and body posture, they can more easily see what feeling we are labeling. It's time to pull out our stage-acting skills.

 What you can say:

- "You look really content after that hug."
- "Wow, I can see you're really excited right now!"
- "Mmm, you seem really frustrated!"
- "Did that make you feel really angry?"
- "All our feelings are okay to feel. Not all behaviors are okay, though."

There are books, cards, and charts, available to print or buy, with different facial expressions labeled with a feeling. We can ask our child to point out which expression best shows how they are feeling and help them label that emotion.

Another way of teaching emotions is by labeling our own feelings. If you have a toddler at home, you may experience a spectrum of emotions on a daily basis from joy, fulfillment, and contentment to frustration, boredom, futility, and anger. Using simple language, we can tell our toddler how we are feeling and point out what we do when we need help regulating our feelings.

 What you can say:

- "I'm feeling really frustrated right now. I'm going to close my eyes and take a really deep breath."

- "I'm feeling very relaxed right now. I really like that I get to spend time with you."
- "I need to take a time-out for a minute because I'm feeling really angry."
- "I am excited that we get to see our friends today."

Emotions are something we feel in the body, and you can teach your child to listen to their body's signals. This can help them process feelings and also help them know when it's important to talk with an adult about something that made them feel unsafe or uncomfortable. Feelings of fear and lack of safety produce a suite of physiological responses, and kids can learn to know when something doesn't feel right. A few of the common physiological responses to fear, anxiety, and lack of safety include

- fast heartbeat
- sick feeling in the tummy or a clenched or tight tummy
- stopping breathing or breathing faster

The first thing we can do toward helping our child recognize these physiological sensations is to ask our child about it. When you notice your child feeling anxious, fearful, or uncomfortable, you can say some of the following things.

 What you can say:

- "Where do you feel that feeling in your body?"
- "Can you put your hand on your body where you have the most feelings right now?"
- "Sometimes when I'm feeling upset, I notice that my stomach feels like a tight knot."

As kids get older and they are able to recognize what's happening in their body, we can teach them that they can listen to this "belly voice." If they ever have a gut feeling that something is not right, they can always go to you for help.

Empathy is a particularly important skill when it comes to relationships. As early as toddlerhood, you can help your child begin to practice empathy and compassion for others and themselves. Just as you teach your child to express their *own* feelings verbally, help children to read facial expressions and identify feelings, such as scared, happy, frustrated, excited, and angry. Charade-style guessing games with expressions are a great way to teach children how to read body language.

 What you can say:

- "I know you wanted that toy, but when you hit Mikey, it hurt him, and he felt very sad."
- "Your brother looks like he's feeling upset right now. Let's ask how we can help."
- "How do you think this person in the picture is feeling?"

A PROACTIVE APPROACH: CREATING TEACHABLE MOMENTS THAT FEEL NATURAL

In addition to recognizing teachable moments that arise naturally, we encourage parents to take a proactive approach to teaching about sexual health. Just as we wouldn't wait for our child to ask about the alphabet, we are doing our child a disservice to wait for them to ask the right questions about sexuality. Instead, through books and toys, you can bring sexual health topics into your home in ways that feel natural. By reading and playing, you are sharing information with your child in different ways and providing more opportunities for questions and discussion. Moreover, having these items in your home helps to normalize discussion around sexual topics.

Books

Reading time with toddlers can be a sweet, calm moment to connect with your child and teach them at the same time. There are now many great kids' books for learning about sexuality. Having several book options available lets kids gravitate to the ones they like best at different stages. Moreover, when a particular situation comes up or kids ask questions, it can sometimes be helpful to be able to say, "Hey, we have a book about that. Let's go get it."

We recommend you get books on various sexuality topics for your child's current age as well as some books appropriate for when they get older. By having books in your home that are suitable for different developmental stages, you will be prepared when your child hits that next stage. (Note that the next stage for your child may be earlier or later than the ages listed in the book.) In our resources sections, you will find a list of a few toddler books we like as well as some good online lists that review books about sexuality for different age groups.

Before you read books about sexuality with your child, *first read them by yourself*. That way, you can decide if there are words or concepts that you want to change or add. Another reason to read these books ahead of time is in case the words or topics cause you discomfort. If that's the case, you will have time to think about your feelings and address them before you sit down for reading time with your child.

Toys and Activities

In addition to books, toys and activities are helpful to have at home. The vast majority of toys sold in the United States do not include even the suggestion of genitalia. We find this quite unfortunate because, again, it turns something normal into a taboo. In the Resources for

Kids section, we list several toys that are anatomically correct. We highly recommend that you have versions of toys with different sexes, regardless of the sex of your child. It's important they learn about differences in anatomy. In addition, dolls can help kids to understand the differences among sex, gender identity, and gender expression.

SUMMARY

- Toddlers are wired for curiosity, so this is a great time to start discussing sexuality.
- Toddlers haven't learned about our cultural norms yet, and they are not self-conscious or inhibited. Although their behaviors might surprise us, it's most likely that your toddler's behaviors and questions represent normal, age-typical behavior.
- When teaching about sexuality, any topic that comes up is fair game. Just make sure to keep your comments short and simple. Common sexuality topics we can teach about include
  - how we value the body and bodily functions
  - accurate names of all body parts
  - reproduction
  - gender
  - feelings
- Subjects that are especially important to teach about are physical boundaries, safety, consent, and privacy. Any time we talk openly about sexuality in a positive way, we are also helping to protect our child.
- A multitude of occasions to teach about sexuality will arise naturally. Do your best to recognize and seize those opportunities. In addition, it's important to be proactive when teaching about sexuality. Appropriate books and toys will go a long way toward helping you do this.

RESOURCES FOR PARENTS

- Educate2Empower Publishing (see https://e2epublishing.info): This publisher offers resources, including books and posters, that you can use at home or in the classroom. Their website includes free resources like the posters "My Body Safety Rules" and "Early Warning Signs" (to help kids identify when they feel unsafe).
- Online booklists:
  - Sex Ed Rescue: https://sexedrescue.com/sex-education-books-for-babies
  - Sex Positive Families: https://sexpositivefamilies.com/resources/reading-list/#infant
  - Colours of Us: https://coloursofus.com/45-multicultural-childrens-books-about-bodies-sex-consent

RESOURCES FOR KIDS

Books

These books are all appropriate for toddlers, and many of them are great to read with your kindergartner too. While it's great to purchase several books to keep in your home, these books are often carried in libraries. If they aren't, ask your local library to purchase them so other families can benefit too! Remember to read them ahead of time to make sure they're right for your family.

ANATOMY

- *Amazing You: Getting Smart About Your Private Parts* by Gail Saltz; Lynne Cravath, Illustrator (Dutton Children's Books)
- *The Bare Naked Book* by Kathy Stinson; Melissa Cho, Illustrator (Annick Press)

- *Who Has What? All About Girls' Bodies and Boys' Bodies* by Robie H. Harris; Nadine Bernard Westcott, Illustrator (Candlewick Press)

BABIES

- *Say Hello to Baby* by Smriti Prasadam-Halls and Britta Teckentrup (Kane Miller Books)

BODIES: HOW THEY WORK, GENERAL

- *Inside Your Outside: All About the Human Body* [The Cat in the Hat's Learning Library®] by Tish Rabe; Aristides Ruiz, Illustrator (Random House)
- *Me and My Amazing Body* by Joan Sweeney; Edward Miller, Illustrator (Alfred A. Knopf)

BODY POSITIVITY

- *Bodies are Cool* by Tyler Feder (Dial Books for Young Readers)
- *Her Body Can* by Katie Crenshaw and Ady Meschke; Li Liu, Illustrator (East 26 Publishing)
- *I Love All of Me* by Lorie Ann Grover; Carolina Búzio, Illustrator (Cartwheel Books)
- *Lovely* by Jess Hong (Creston Books)
- *Toot* by Leslie Patricelli (Candlewick Press)

BOUNDARIES AND CONSENT

- *A Hug* by Nicola Manton; Magali Garcia, Illustrator (self-published)
- *Ask First, Monkey! A Playful Introduction to Consent and Boundaries* by Juliet Clare Bell; Abigail Tompkins, Illustrator (Jessica Kingsley Publishers)

- *Can I Give You a Squish?* by Emily Neilson (Penguin Random House)
- *Miles Is the Boss of His Body* by Abbie Schiller and Samantha Kurtzman-Counter (The Mother Company)
- *No Means No! Teaching Personal Boundaries, Respect and Consent; Empowering Kids by Respecting Their Choices and Their Right to Say, "No!"* by Jayneen Sanders; Cherie Zamazing, Illustrator (Educate2Empower Publishing)
- *Will Ladybug Hug?* by Hilary Leung (Scholastic)

BOUNDARIES AND CONSENT FOR ATYPICAL KIDS

- *An Exceptional Children's Guide to Touch: Teaching Social and Physical Boundaries to Kids* by Hunter Manasco; Katharine Manasco, Illustrator (Jessica Kingsley Publishers)

FAMILIES

- *And Tango Makes Three* by Justin Richardson and Peter Parnell; Henry Cole, Illustrator (Simon & Schuster Books for Young Readers)
- *The Family Book* by Todd Parr (Little, Brown and Company)
- *Heather Has Two Mommies* by Lesléa Newman; Laura Cornell, Illustrator (Candlewick Press)
- *Just the Way We Are* by Jessica Shirvington and Claire Robertson (ABC Books)
- *Stella Brings the Family* by Miriam B. Schiffer; Holly Clifton-Brown, Illustrator (Chronicle Books)
- *Two Is Enough* by Janna Matthies; Tuesday Mourning, Illustrator (RP Kids)
- *Who's In My Family? All About Our Families* by Robie H. Harris; Nadine Bernard Westcott, Illustrator (Candlewick Press)

FEELINGS

- *In My Heart: A Book of Feelings* by Jo Witek; Christine Roussey, Illustrator (Abrams Appleseed)
- *Lots of Feelings* by Shelley Rotner (Millbrook Press)
- *My Body Sends a Signal: Helping Kids Recognize Emotions and Express Feelings* by Natalia Maguire; Anastasia Zababashkina, Illustrator (Maguire Books)
- *The Feelings Series* [10-book collection; any books in this series] by Trace Moroney (Five Mile/Regency Media)
- *You, Me and Empathy: Teaching Children About Empathy, Feelings, Kindness, Compassion, Tolerance and Recognising Bullying Behaviours* by Jayneen Sanders; Sofia Cardoso, Illustrator (Educate2Empower Publishing)

GENDER

- *Annie's Plaid Shirt* by Stacy B. Davids; Rachael Balsaitis and Sam Pines, Illustrators (Upswing Press)
- *Introducing Teddy: A Gentle Story About Gender and Friendship* by Jessica Walton; Dougal MacPherson, Illustrator (Bloomsbury)
- *No Difference Between Us: Teaching Children About Gender Equality, Respectful Relationships, Feelings, Choice, Self-Esteem, Empathy, Tolerance, and Acceptance* by Jayneen Sanders; Amanda Gulliver, Illustrator (Educate2Empower Publishing)
- *Red: A Crayon's Story* by Michael Hall (Greenwillow Books)

REPRODUCTION

- *The Science of Babies: A Little Book for Big Questions About Bodies, Birth, and Families* by Deborah Roffman; Frank Cable, Illustrator (Birdhouse)
- *What Makes a Baby* by Cory Silverberg; Fiona Smyth, Illustrator (Seven Stories Press)

- *What's in There? All About Before You Were Born* by Robie H. Harris; Nadine Bernard Westcott, Illustrator (Candlewick Press)
- *What's the Big Secret? Talking About Sex With Girls and Boys* by Laurie Krasny Brown and Mark Brown (Little, Brown and Co.)
- *Where Do Babies Come From? Usborne Lift-the-Flap First Questions and Answers* by Katie Daynes (Usborne Books)

Toys and Activities

Dolls, games, and other activities are a great idea for introducing, reinforcing, and normalizing sexuality concepts. These work best when you play *with* your child. As you interact, you can answer questions and provide information proactively.

DOLLS

- In Europe: Paola Reina®
- In the United States: Miniland®

GAMES AND ACTIVITIES

- Hape/Beleduc® Your Body 5-Layer Wooden Puzzle. The puzzle comes in four versions: boy, girl, woman with baby, and man.
- Janod® Emotions Magnetic Game
- Melissa & Doug® Magnetic Human Body Play Set. You can use this set to discuss the different aspects of sexual identity. For example, talk about the difference between biological sex and gender identity.
- Todd Parr Feelings Flash Cards

SONG/VIDEO

- Teeny Tiny Stevies, *Boss of My Own Body*, YouTube video: https://www.youtube.com/watch?v=nLpjNJnXZlU

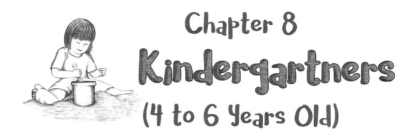

Chapter 8
Kindergartners
(4 to 6 Years Old)

If you are feeling concern about starting to read this book now—when your child is kindergarten age—rather than earlier, don't worry! Regardless of the age of your child, learning about sexual health benefits you, your child, and your relationship with them. It isn't too late to start. Even if your child is already 5 or 6 years old, the content of this book is relevant. If your child is already 7 years old or older, the information in this book can be helpful along with books specifically geared toward older children (you can find a list in the Resources for Parents and Resources for Kids sections in Chapter 10).

Exploding linguistic capacity coupled with substantial cognitive gains and cultural awareness allow children in the kindergarten years to engage in and talk about elements of life (including sexuality) in increasingly complex and interesting ways. It is still very useful to have a solid handle on the ways that things were explained during the toddler years—so, if you haven't read Chapter 7, go back and have a quick read through. The information and suggestions here reference and build on those toddler experiences. They remain good starting places for a 4- to 6-year-old child who didn't receive that scaffolding during their toddler years.

In addition to cognitive and verbal development, the other substantial growth for kindergartners is their social development. They are able to understand and participate in social interactions and moral judgments in new and engaging ways. During these years, they often experience novel social connections and learning outside of the family unit. They learn about other sets of cultures, values, and perspectives from their friends and peers in preschool, kindergarten, and first grade. Media also has a growing role in informing and molding kindergartners' understanding of bodies, relationships, identities, and boundaries.

Parents by and large continue to have primary control over many influential elements of their children's learning about relationships and sexual health at this time. They are able to choose a preschool and may even have flexibility over the kindergarten their child attends. They are able to choose whether, how much, and to what specific media content their children have access to at home. They can expose their child to values, morals, and stories of their families. Children in this age range continue to find much pleasure in imitating the adults around them, although not always in the ways that the adults want to be imitated!

Parents sometimes feel overwhelmed by the process of deciding on the inputs of peers and media in their children's lives. But you do have this kind of control at this age. If children ask questions (and kindergartners are known for asking challenging questions!), you can answer honestly and say that, for example, in your family, you go to church every weekend, or you don't watch movies, or you spend Friday nights watching movies together, or you wait until you're teenagers to wear two-piece bathing suits. If discerning your values is an ongoing process for you, you can also be honest with your child about that. Let your child know that you're learning more and thinking more and have decided that some family rules may change as a result.

We recommend that kindergartners' digital media usage be kept to a minimum. While we know that many parents either choose to give their children access to media or have a need for media to entertain their child at times, research is clear that very low levels of media are best for children's development (Council on Communications and Media et al., 2016). The reason is that children benefit substantially from active engagement with the adults in their lives—and media tends to reduce rather than increase active engagement. Additionally, children who use media without consistent, active engagement with their parents have increased risks of viewing adult content or other negative imagery (Radesky & Christakis, 2016).

Children in this age range rarely seek out sexual content online. Therefore, using parental controls can *reduce* the chances of them coming across problematic videos and other imagery. However, as children become more curious and start to use words (like *sex*) that are often poorly defined, they may go to the internet to search for answers. At this age, children do not need to have access to search engines. When children start searching for information about sex and sexuality online, it becomes increasingly difficult for parental controls to be effective. Further, in the online space, people who want to harm children look for unsupervised children. Although these predators are less common than you might believe them to be, they are still present, and it is critical to take them into account when considering what internet safety is for your child.

Start a conversation about internet safety with your child as soon as they begin to have access to media without your direct participation. Let them know that the internet has things that are for adults, by adults, and can make children feel yucky. Let them know that if they ever come across something that makes them feel yucky, you are able to help them. Let them know you will never be upset with them for anything that they share with you.

HOW KINDERGARTNERS ARE LEARNING

Like toddlers, kindergartners learn through

- community,
- expression,
- identity,
- independence,
- media,
- nature,
- patterns,
- peers,
- play,
- story,
- their bodies, and
- wonder.

This is a long list of ways that children in this age range learn. Here, we highlight (in bold) a few of these ways that kindergartners learn and how those learning formats intersect with sex and sexuality, both now and in the future (EL Education, n.d.).

Children learn through **expression** by trying out different expressions themselves, including facial, verbal, gender, and so many more. This is essentially the child sharing what it feels like and means to be them and to feel positively about themselves when others are able to understand them. The feedback loop that comes with expression is a powerful learning tool: Peers, parents, other family members, teachers, and even with strangers may comment on and try to engage with children. These reactions provide information about what is culturally and socially appropriate and how the child is expected to act in a wide range of scenarios (Cacciatore et al., 2020).

Children learn through **media** by connecting and integrating what they see and hear in movies, songs, advertisements, and YouTube videos as well as on social media, the computer, and phone games with their real-life experiences. This intersection of influences and considerations of what is good and healthy to engage with can be potentially problematic. Parents retain immense potential for influence, control, and ultimately framing of digital content with children in this age group. Karen had a parent reach out to her for advice on how to prevent their 4-year-old from viewing porn. The problem was easily resolved when the parent removed the computer from the child's room. While the solution in this situation feels very evident, the fact is that parents of 4- to 6-year-olds always play a huge role in mediating the media-based experiences of their children, and doing so can have profoundly positive effects (Nobre et al., 2020).

Finding **patterns** (another way that kindergartners learn!) sometimes happens a little more quickly when a parent points out these little connections. Learning bodily care, and putting a priority on that over immediate fun, establishes clear lines to taking responsible steps with one's body and the bodies of one's partners much later in life. One way we see children this age recognizing patterns is in their propensity toward black-and-white terms and overgeneralized rules. Because they are just learning cultural constructs, they want to show mastery of them and indicate that they are part of the larger cultural circle. So, they often separate themselves into single-gender groups and desire adherence to gender norms as part of acceptance into those groups.

Children learn from their **peers** in preschool, school, church, playgroups, and any other setting where they engage with other similar-aged children. These influences can bring knowledge of sexuality in ways that are supportive of and/or different from home-based messages. Being highly engaged with your child's friends and encouraging delving into whatever conversation topics they bring home allow you to consider the messages your child is getting from their peers and provide connects or disconnection from your family's approach.

For example, a great time to reinforce your family values would be if your child tells you a story about playing house with their friends at school and that one friend said their play family couldn't have two fathers. You could remind your child of a family friend who has two fathers, tell a story about someone you know who is part of a two-father household, or read a children's book together about such a situation.

Children learn through **play** by reenacting what they see and experience in the world around them. Kids inform each other and learn from each other about what is possible in each of their family units; thus, they expand their own smaller worlds into a larger collective. One of Karen's friends overheard a mixed-gender group of children on a playground playing house and arguing about who would be the mother. One of the children in the group had lesbian parents. She informed the group with firmness and gravitas that a household could have two mothers. The children all nodded along—most of them knew her parents. A boy asked if there could be two fathers. The girl looked at him and said, "I don't know anything about that!" This interaction both informed the children and also expanded their curiosity. Other examples of the ways that kindergarten-aged children learn through play is playing doctor and looking at other children's genitals or pretending to be dating or married (including holding hands and kissing). All are developmentally expected behaviors at this age.

Children learn through **their bodies** by trying something out and seeing how it feels. Children who are able to make mistakes like falling, tripping, or running into something learn what those things feel like to their bodies and then make adjustments in the future. They are also able to learn what feels good to their bodies. Children of all ages may explore their body, touching every part of it to understand what that part does. When this includes touching their genitals, parents may be surprised. However, this is entirely developmentally expected. In some situations in which kids are learning their body, it is helpful to have an adult present to assist them in seeing the bigger picture. For example, learning about body care and doing something that may be considered boring—like brushing your teeth—can become a standard part of a morning and evening routine with an adult who can ask questions like, "How do

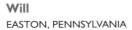

Will
EASTON, PENNSYLVANIA

Father to two children
Age when first child was born: 30

I took Ryan to the park when he was about 4 years old. He climbed the stairs to the slide and spent a lot of time at the top of the slide. Thinking he was nervous, I encouraged him to slide, assuring him I would be there to catch him. Eventually, he rode down the slide, and as he jumped into my arms, he said, "Daddy, what does *fuck* mean?" Apparently, he was not nervous at the top of the slide; he was just reading the graffiti.

Even though I am more equipped than most to answer such a question, this was earlier than expected. I stumbled my way through the best age-appropriate answer I could give, mindful of the possible ramifications of his repeating the word to other children and adults. I remember that part of my lesson was that it was a word that made a lot of adults very anxious, especially when they heard it spoken by a young child. He observed that it was weird for adults to fuss over a word, and I had to agree.

A few years later, my fears would resurface. Ryan included an (entirely accurate) discussion of sex in one of his projects in first grade. His teacher, unprepared for such a submission, told him his work was "inappropriate," and he felt ashamed. I reached out to other adults in our lives, and they wrote him letters, offering their support for his artwork. It totally changed his feelings, and he wasn't ashamed anymore!

your teeth feel after you've brushed them compared to before you've brushed them?"

The thing to take away from this discussion is that kindergartners are always learning, through a multitude of different processes, soaking up information and guidance from the world around them in sophisticated and long-lasting ways. Use one or more of the ways children in this age group learn—see the earlier list—to connect with your kindergartner when you are trying to teach or engage them on any specific sexuality-related content.

WHAT KINDERGARTNERS ARE LEARNING

An important thing to keep in mind about conversations about sex and sexuality is that the larger, overarching topics are essentially the same across the lifespan. What changes are the specific messages and information that come at each age, how deeply the topics are explored, and how the information relates to the current or future sexuality, or both, of the child. Therefore, the age-appropriate information here generally repeats and then expands on the content presented in the toddler chapter (see Chapter 7). If you are just starting with intentional conversations with your child, be sure to backtrack to the conversations in that chapter before diving into the ones that follow.

Bodies

The early years of life center on figuring out how to move in and be in control of one's body. By the time a child is 5 or 6, they are ready to integrate the immediate physicality of the first few years into their increasingly cognitive understanding of themselves and the world around them.

BODY ACCEPTANCE

Children as young as kindergarten may already have concerns about their body and feel judgment from their peers, their family, and the media about the way that it looks and works. Finding ways to shift negative or judgmental assessments and comparisons of their bodies to neutral or open descriptions can set up a lifetime of body acceptance.

 What you can say:

- "Yes, that child in your group is really tall. Isn't it cool that all our bodies grow differently?"
- "I know your friend can't swim yet, but everyone learns things at different times, and that's okay."
- "No, you're not as fast. I can see why that would be frustrating for you. But, everybody's body is different. What is something that your body does really well?"

HUMOR

The childhood fascination with bodies and all of their weird shapes, sensations, methods of elimination, and sounds only increases as kids hit kindergarten age. Pee, poop, and genitalia become elements of an amazing array of toilet humor. Fart jokes are the pinnacle of collective hilarity. All of this humor comes, essentially, from engagement and interest in how the body that they are living in works, from connecting with their peers on matters that are surprising and highly personal to their lived experience. While most adults are somewhat less interested in toilet humor than kindergartners, it benefits your relationship with your child to find ways to laugh together. This also allows you to draw a line when the location or the topic of their humor becomes truly inappropriate, offensive, or insulting. Our children are more able to hear us when we guide them away from some kinds of humor when we do participate with their humor other times.

What you can say:

- "That joke's hilarious!"
- "Hahahahaha!"
- "This joke is actually more hurtful than funny. Let me share why . . ."

Allegra
BROOKLYN PARK, MINNESOTA

Mother to two children
Age when first child was born: 29

Today, I was downstairs putting away some laundry while Violet and Stella played upstairs in their room. I could tell they were also in my walk-in closet because I heard them clomping around on the wooden floor in some of my high heels. Happy to let them play, I kept on working. All of a sudden, I hear 4 ½-year-old Violet say, "Mommy, we found the most amazing thing! Come see!" I told her I was almost done with the laundry, and I'd be up soon. Then I hear little Stella yelling, "Mama, mama! Come see our scissor hat!"

Your scissor hat? Huh?

I go upstairs, and the door to the walk-in closet is closed. Violet yells out, "She didn't say scissor hat, she said SISTER hat—and look!"

Then the door flings open, and the two come out, one cup of my favorite bra gently cupping each of their heads, their outside arm each through one of the arm holes, and the back strap buckled near their chins. They proceed to sashay around the room, telling me about the "amazing sister hat where sisters who are friends can be together forever!"

Life could be a lot worse than sweetness like that.

Internal Anatomy

This is a great time to start talking with kids about internal reproductive anatomy in addition to external. Kindergartners are able to understand things they can't actually see and how two-dimensional representations can depict three-dimensional realities. Books and other two-dimensional imagery of anatomy and reproduction are great helpers to support this process. (Our book recommendations for this age group are at the end of this chapter.)

What you can say:
- "Remember how we've been talking about babies growing inside a uterus? Let's look at a picture in this book to see where it actually is."
- "Remember how your pee comes out of the urethra? It's held in the bladder, which is just a little bit inside and up above your pelvic bone."

Reproduction

Many kindergartners ask questions that so many parents dread: "How does the sperm get inside the uterus and fallopian tubes? How does it get from inside one person's body to inside another person's body?" (If this question has not come up by the time a child is 7 or so, it's important for the parent to bring it up!)

Many parents have reservations about telling their child about reproduction and especially about sexual intercourse as a precursor to pregnancy. Many parents are simply uncomfortable with the idea of talking about how penile–vaginal sex works. We get it. Talking about sex and sexuality can feel uncomfortable, even among adults.

When it comes to teaching about reproduction, we—Laura and Karen—often hear two big concerns from parents, and both are specifically related to teaching about sexual intercourse. One concern parents have is that teaching kids about penile–vaginal sex will ruin their innocence. We believe that it is harmful to a child's

Billie
DAVIS, CALIFORNIA

Aunt and coparent to two children
Age when first became a coparent: 35

When Mia was about 5 years old, she came to me with questions about her vagina. I didn't know how to respond. She knew that her body parts were different from her brother's but didn't know why. One day, Mia asked me why her 'gina hurt. "What?!" I asked, fearing the worst. "Why do you think it is hurting you?" Mia shrugged. "Sometimes, my 'gina can hurt," she answered, pointing to her crotch.

"Does it hurt a lot?" She shook her head. "Only when I press down on it. Does yours ever hurt?" "Sometimes," I answered. I wasn't sure if this was the right time to talk about menstrual cycles and cramps. "They can be really sensitive sometimes, depending on what we eat or if I'm sick." "So, everyone's 'ginas can hurt?" I nodded, answering, "Well, everyone is different, but our bodies can all hurt in different ways." "And boys 'ginas hurt too?" I chuckled, "Yes, they can, especially if they get hurt in that area, too, like if there's punching or hitting. But they don't have vaginas, they have penises."

Mia thought about that for a few seconds and then tried to do the splits. "When I do this, it sometimes hurts." "Oh, darling. I see. Then maybe don't do that when it hurts. Or, maybe we can stretch our legs and get our bodies ready for when we want to exercise." Mia smiled, "That sounds like fun." "Yeah, it can be!" "So, nothing is wrong with me?" "NO! Of course not, darling. But it's very good that you came to talk to me to let me know." We went back to practicing some stretching.

innocence when they learn about sex in a way that is shocking or upsetting for them. Your child *will* learn about sex. If we teach our child about it ourselves, we can infuse the lesson with all the good feelings and values we want them to associate with it. We can explain that sex is for consenting adults only. We can discuss what a miracle birth and life are, and we can discuss sex in the context of our values. Although the information about sex needs to be factual, we are not just talking about the "plumbing." We are talking about our values at the same time.

A second concern parents have is that telling children about sex will implicitly give them permission to do it or that they'll want to try it out. In fact, youths who receive comprehensive sexual health education are more likely to delay sexual activities themselves (Breuner et al., 2016; Ramírez-Villalobos et al., 2021). We encourage parents to give kids context whenever they discuss this topic with their young child. Explicitly state that sexual activities are for grown-ups who both agree they want to do it. If you've been teaching your child about boundaries around genitalia—that only they should be touching their own genitals (with few exceptions)—that knowledge will help to clarify that sex is only for adults.

Florence

AMSTERDAM, THE NETHERLANDS

Mother to two children
Age when first child was born: 40

I'm pretty open with my kids about sexuality, so when my daughter was 4, she had known for a while that a baby is made when an egg from one person gets together with the sperm of another person. And she knew that a baby grows in a uterus. I thought I had the reproduction topic covered with as much detail as I needed to tell her for now. What else does a 4-year-old need to know? And then one night she asked, "How does the sperm *get* to the egg?" Gulp! I was *not* prepared for this conversation. But I decided now was the right time to start talking. She had asked about it, and we were in a good situation for talking while snuggling before her bedtime.

(continues)

(continued)

> I calmed my voice and told her that there are some different ways the egg and sperm can get together. I said something like,
>
>> One way is that a person with a penis and a person with a vagina can fit the penis and vagina together. Then a bunch of little sperm all wiggle out of the penis, through the vagina and the uterus, and into these tubes called fallopian tubes. Then the sperm just kind of hang out and wait for an egg to come. If an egg comes, it gets to choose which sperm it lets in. Then the egg with the sperm goes back to the uterus, and that's where the baby grows.
>
> I paused to see her reaction, and she seemed interested. So then I told her,
>
>> Sometimes a doctor gets the sperm from one person and uses a little medical instrument to put the sperm in the uterus of another person. Other times, a doctor can get the sperm and egg and put them together in a laboratory, and then they are put into a person's uterus when they are already together. Isn't that amazing?
>
> At age 4, I felt this was a good beginning and patted myself on the back. It wasn't until a year later during my fourth conversation with her about intercourse that she got it. She was now 5 years old, and we were reading a new children's book about sexuality. There was an illustration of two people in bed under the covers and a description of what they were doing. I read it to her, and with wide eyes, she said, "That's how it happens?!" I had to smile. By this point, I had gotten past my jitters over the topic, and I made sure to reiterate it's only for adults and not something that kids do.

PUBERTY

In kindergarten, children rarely have personal connections to elements of puberty, but they are able to understand that process, which makes it a great time to start talking about it in concrete, specific terms. Because all of the pubertal changes are years away, children are able to learn the information as purely information rather than as imminent and very personal (and potentially unwelcome) changes to their own bodies. It gives them years to think over and prepare themselves for the changes, rather than being surprised to learn about those changes as they are happening to them or their peers.

 What you can say:

- "You're right. I have pubic hair, and you don't. You'll grow more hair all over your body, but especially your pubic area, underarms, legs, and face, when your body grows from a kid's body to an adult's body. That's called *puberty*, and it usually starts at some point between the ages of 8 and 14 years old."
- "Periods are something that most people with a uterus start when they're around 12. I was (how old you were) years old when I started mine. You might start your period a little earlier or a little later, but it will probably be around that time. I'll be there to help you whenever it happens!"

Social Identity

Kindergartners are beginning to understand the social context that they live in and how it relates to themselves, their families, and their friends. Explicit conversations about identity-related elements help children learn to navigate complexities with skill and finesse.

GENDER

Research about gender has made it clear that children are often acutely aware of gender norms and stereotypes by this age (Chung & Huang, 2021). That includes children whose gender identity does not align with the sex they were assigned at birth, who often, although not always, express their gender identity by this age (Schaad, 2022). For children who identify as trans or nonbinary, making room for this identity questioning and development is a critical piece of effective parenting (Katz-Wise et al., 2022).

Many children will go through a time when they want to use a nickname, try out different clothes, and engage with a range of toy and identity options. When parents are open to this exploration, children may or may not migrate back to the gender identity associated with their sex assigned at birth while feeling increasingly connected to their parents. When parents stop children from exploring their identities, they are teaching their child that they will only accept the child within a narrow range of identities and behaviors, which has a long-term negative impact on the relationship (Pullen Sansfaçon et al., 2020; Sansfaçon et al., 2018). This is, in many ways, a precursor to the adolescent years, when personal identity consideration becomes even more present in young people's daily lives and interactions with their families.

Melissa
ASHEVILLE, NORTH CAROLINA

Mother to two children
Age when first child was born: 29

I'm so proud of River. He came running home to say that a girl he just met didn't believe he's a boy (given his name, his two French braids, and his "girl" clothing). She asked to see his penis to "prove he's a boy." He didn't show her, even though she flashed her private parts at him multiple times. I guess she was "showing him hers" to inspire him to do the same. But he came straight home from the neighbors' house and told me! I'm proud of him for holding his boundary and coming to me, rather than showing his private parts to a random kid!

I think I handled it okay. First, I validated him not needing to show her anything and said I was glad he came straight to me to tell me about it. He was quite offended by the situation ("Why won't she just believe I'm a boy if I say so?!"), but he also really liked the girl and wanted to continue to play with her. He didn't want to go back and play, though, unless I talked to her so she would stop making a big deal about it.

Talking to her felt like a big step since I don't know her or her parents, but I asked him to call her over to meet me. We had a sweet initial conversation about how amazing it is that she could be so much taller than him when he's actually a month older. Then, I gently mentioned that River had told me she didn't believe he's a boy and that she'd shown him her private parts and asked to see his. I said, "You're not in trouble, but I just want to know if that's true." She glanced sideways at him and blushed a little, but said, "Yes." I asked if her parents had ever told her not to show her private parts to people outside their family, and she again said, "Yes."

I said, "Good! Thank you for being honest. I just wanted to be sure you knew it's not a good idea to pull your underwear down in front of other people, or to ask anyone else to do that either." I continued, "There can be tricky people out there, and we want all kids to be safe and to feel comfortable with their privacy. Does that make sense?" She again blushed a little and said, "Yes," and I switched back to talk about how much fun they were having and that if they were having fun and being safe and kind, it really didn't matter what kind of genitalia they each had.

She got it, and they ran back to play some more—where I could see them—and I felt a rush of relief at having navigated a potentially tricky moment with relative grace!

 What you can say:

- "If you want to try out a nickname that's different from your name, we can talk about it. The most important thing is that your name is really about you feeling more like yourself rather than trying to be more like someone else."
- "So many different colors and shapes of clothes are fun! You can try on a bunch of different things and tell us what feels best on your body."

FAMILY DYNAMICS

Kindergartners are increasingly interested and engaged in their peers' families and how they're organized. The ultimate question here is, Who lives at home? Two parents? One parent and a grandparent? Four or five older or younger siblings? Aunt, uncles, or cousins? How were these families built? Through adoption, fostering, intercourse, surrogacy, or IVF?

For an increasing portion of families, this conversation about family configuration includes elements of identities. If there are two parents in a household, is it a mother and a father or two mothers or two fathers, or is at least one of the parents nonbinary? Or are there two mothers and two fathers? In one of the families that Karen knows, the four parents are all gay and intentionally coparenting together. But in other families, it might be a heterosexual couple that divorced and both remarried, or a gay couple that divorced and both remarried. Another family Karen knows has three mothers and one father: a lesbian couple and a heterosexual couple; one of the lesbians and the father were the original parents. Karen and Laura also know children who are being raised by grandparents, either as a coparent with three generations in the household or as the sole caregiver of a child. Having parents who are able to provide a place where their children can come home and ask questions and discuss these elements of family structure is critical to helping them navigate the complex world they live in.

 What you can say:

- "Because there are all kinds of people in the world, families are made in all kinds of different ways. Let's talk about your family: Who is in your family? Do you know the relationships between all of those people?"
- "What are some of the different kinds of families your friends have? Do they have the same number of siblings and parents as you, or are they different? What do you think might be good about those ways of being a family? What do you think is good about our way of being a family?"

The thing you will notice about these conversations so far is that they are deeply steeped in cultural expectations. They help kindergartners consider and think about the world around them. It opens up a conversation space between you and your child that provides opportunities for you to continue talking throughout childhood and into adolescence and adulthood. This is the case with many topics around this age. The other thing we want to highlight is body image.

Allegra
BROOKLYN PARK, MINNESOTA

Mother to two children
Age when first child was born: 29

Well, sign me up. After today, the family might end up on *The Maury Povich Show* or *The Jerry Springer Show*. Not my plan. I want to be on Oprah on one of her "Favorite Things" days!

A few weeks ago, Violet came home and told me that since the kids in her preschool class are going to kindergarten in a few weeks, they did a "my future" project, where their teacher interviewed them about their dreams for the future and videotaped it. Violet was so excited for me to see it. Today, we got an email with a link to the video and a request from the teachers to not be driving, doing important tasks like surgery, or drinking anything while we were watching. A few minutes in, I could see why.

Many of the kids had some pretty side-slapping answers to the questions, such as these: "When I grow up, I want to rip out people's teeth, like my mom does" (she's a dentist) and "When I grow up, I want to be older, but not as old as a mummy like my dad." But Violet's took the cake. Here is her answer to one of the questions, verbatim: "When I grow up, I am going to either marry my little sister and live in a cabin in the mountains or live alone forever with hundreds of cats."

Like I said, daytime TV talk show, here we come.

Feelings

What kindergartners are learning about feelings will last them a lifetime. These early habits around feelings form the basis for the ways that children, and then teenagers, and then adults, and then older adults navigate the emotional landscape. Ideally, children are invited to experience their feelings in a nonjudgmental environment, consider what their feelings are, talk about how to understand them, locate the feelings in their bodies, and talk with people they love and trust about these details, their causes, and their resolutions.

 What you can say:

- "I see your face is all scrunched up. Are you having a strong feeling?"
- "Is there a word that describes how your body feels right now?"
- "It's okay to not know how you're feeling. Can I ask you some questions about what's happening in your stomach, your head, and your chest to help us figure it out together?"
- "Let's think back together about what happened right before you started feeling this way. Do you remember?"

Incorporating these elements of emotional intelligence into the natural flow of conversation in the home allows it to feel like an integrating bridge between a child's growing experience of their internal and external world. It sets them on a path of health, appropriate self-analysis, and conversations with others that will support their relationships for their entire lives. Incorporating an emotions chart that has simple pictures of people's faces having different emotions can be helpful.

Body Boundaries and Consent

Kindergartners are often deeply righteous. Because of their adherence to rules and a desire for everything to fit neatly into a specific part of a rigid pattern, kindergartners who learn about boundaries and consent become consent's best advocates. Kindergartners are also at an age at which they are learning about friendship connections that reach far beyond side-by-side play. For the first time, they are learning about the complexities of peer-to-peer negotiation about physical space, coveted items, and types of play and other ways to spend time.

Moreover, children in this age group are naturally curious about others' bodies and genitals, and many have not yet developed a sense of self-consciousness or embarrassment. As a result, time with peers can be exploratory. Children may want to see their peers' genitals, compare them, or touch them. If this occurs, we—Laura and Karen—hope that the adults in the situation will respond without shaming the children involved. We parents want to teach appropriate boundaries and, at the same time, recognize that these types of situations between similar-aged peers are most often displays of typical curiosity. (In Chapter 9, we discuss strategies for how to respond to surprising situations. Teachers can also benefit from this information.) Teaching your child appropriate boundaries at home as well as supporting them when they set physical boundaries with others can help your child avoid inappropriate behavior at school or tell you if it happens.

 What you can say:

- "You and your friend have different ideas about what to do next. What questions can you ask each other to understand what they want?"
- "How can you tell someone that you don't want a hug? What could you do if they didn't listen to you?"
- "You don't have to share all of your things with your friend. It is important to keep your really special things just for you to play with. But it is important to figure out what you can share. Can you pick five things to play with your friend when they come over?"

Privacy

Children in this age range are often experiencing (or they are watching their friends experience) their first desires for privacy. Their growing body awareness coupled with their increasing cultural awareness bring children in this age to request time away from their parents for the first time. For example, they may ask to change clothes, bathe, or use the toilet alone. When parents are able to provide their children with the physical and emotional space to access privacy, they are teaching that the child's desire for autonomy is valid and something that they can and should expect from other relationships in the future.

 What you can say:

- "If you'd like to be alone for your shower, that's totally fine! I'll leave the door cracked so you can call for me if you need help with anything."
- "You can always choose to get dressed by yourself, but you do have to remember that when it's cold outside to choose pants!"

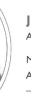

Judith
AMSTERDAM, THE NETHERLANDS

Mother to two children
Age when first child was born: 22

When I asked Juno to get dressed this morning, she picked out her own clothes and put them on, just like I asked . . . in front of the window with the curtains open. She didn't even think about the fact that any of the people living across our street might see her.

I was so prudish at that age. I remember trying to get my swimsuit on at the beach. It must have been one of the greatest challenges of my childhood, wrapping my towel around me to hide my body away from anyone who might see me. Of course, standing in the sand on one leg while trying to get the other one in the right hole of my bathing suit was nearly impossible, and during the summer, I had to do that multiple times a week. Juno doesn't bother with any of that stuff. She just takes off her clothes, sits down on her towel, and puts on her swimsuit. She doesn't care at all that anyone might see her.

Last summer, she was swimming naked almost every day in our vacation pool in France. She looked free as a bird. I wonder when she will start closing the curtains, or if she ever will.

Maya
AMSTERDAM, THE NETHERLANDS

Mother to one child
Age when child was born: 41

Chloe has been doing this thing lately that sort of confuses me. On the one hand, she has been increasingly private about being naked and sometimes even asks me to leave the room when she is changing. (And she definitely wants a towel around her so no one can see her change out of her suit at the pool.) But then, on the other hand, she seems very interested in overtly showing her private parts to Mike and me.

Lately, Chloe has even had this phase where she'll ask me to interact with her and, for instance, "sniff her butthole." Even when I tell her I won't because I don't want to, and it's not so nice, she makes a joke out of it and seems really insistent that I put my nose there because "it would feel funny." Another time, after the shower, she lay down on the floor while I was still drying her off, and a strand of my hair touched her vulva. She said, "Mommy do that again. It feels really nice!" It is really confusing to me how to respond to those things. I do not want her to feel bad or ashamed for having the urge, but, obviously, I also do not want to comply! So far, I have just told her that "yes, that feels funny, but it is only for you, yourself, to interact with."

SUMMARY

- Kindergarten-aged children are learning through a wide range of means: community, expression, identity, independence, media, nature, play, peers, rhythm, story, their bodies, patterns, and wonder. Parents still have a fair amount of control over many of these elements, being able to choose, for example, what media their children consume in the home environment. Some of these elements are less readily controlled, like peers. However, parents can still engage with their children at home, discuss and consider information and perspectives that peers bring, and reiterate parental and home-based values.
- In addition to learning through a wide range of media, kindergarten-aged children are also learning about many different topics related to sexuality. Regarding their bodies, children this age have moved on from the basics to things like body acceptance, appropriate (and inappropriate!) body-related humor, internal anatomy, reproduction, and puberty. Regarding their identities and their places in the world, children this age are considering gender, family dynamics, feelings, appropriate physical boundaries, consent, and privacy. Taken together, these elements of the physical self and how it can or should or shouldn't connect with other people's physical selves is a huge step in emotional and social growth.

RESOURCES FOR PARENTS

As the discussion around supporting healthy sexuality during early childhood grows, more and more resources become available to help us parents along. We have provided some great ones here. Any videos intended for children to watch should be watched along with a caregiver the first few times. If used wisely, kids' videos can be a great resource. Watch them on your own first. If you like them, they will reinforce the messages you are sending and will also be an opportunity to continue your ongoing dialogue about sexuality with your child.

Online Programs, Videos, and Podcasts

- AMAZE Jr. resources for parents and videos for kids: https://amaze.org/jr
- *Amy Lang's Just Say This!* audio podcast: https://birdsandbeesandkids.com/category/podcast
- Common Sense Media, which offers comprehensive reviews of media, such as videos and movies, as well as information on how to use parental controls: https://www.commonsensemedia.org
- Unitarian Universalist Association, which offers world-renowned, fact-based sexual health education programs called Our Whole Lives (or OWL); for parents and caregivers of children in kindergarten and first grade, the association also offers an excellent list of resources and short videos: https://www.uua.org/re/owl/videos-k-1

Online Booklists

- Sex Ed Rescue: https://sexedrescue.com/sex-education-books-for-children/#ages
- Sex Positive Families: https://sexpositivefamilies.com/resources/reading-list/#school
- Colours of Us: https://coloursofus.com/45-multicultural-childrens-books-about-bodies-sex-consent

RESOURCES FOR KIDS

In addition to the resources listed here, those listed for toddlers (see Chapter 7) are also still mostly interesting and enjoyable for kindergartners, especially if they are not yet familiar with them.

Books

Here we have listed many of our favorite books for kindergartners. Like the books we mentioned for toddlers, there are a lot of good books available. Read them on your own first. In addition, encourage your public library to carry them. That way, you can have more sexuality books in your rotation, spend less money on them, and make them available for other kids in your neighborhood. (If you're so inclined, many libraries will also take new books as a donation. If possible, it's a great way to support your community!)

ANATOMY

- *Your Whole Body: From Your Head to Your Toes, and Everything in Between!* by Lizzie DeYoung Charbonneau; Misha Iver, Illustrator (Arctic Flower Publishing)

BABIES

- *Hello Benny! What It's Like to Be a Baby* by Robie H. Harris; Michael Emberley, Illustrator (Margaret K. McElderry Books)

HOW BODIES WORK, GENERAL

- *Human Body Theater: A Non-Fiction Revue* by Maris Wicks (First Second)
- *The Magic School Bus: Inside the Human Body* by Joanna Cole; Bruce Degen, Illustrator (Scholastic)
- *Professor Astro Cat's Human Body Odyssey* by Dominic Walliman; Ben Newman, Illustrator (Flying Eye Books)
- *The Usborne Flip-Flap Body Book* by Alastair Smith and Judy Tatchell; Maria Wheatley, Illustrator (Usborne)

BODY POSITIVITY

- *All Bodies Are Good Bodies* by Charlotte Barkla; Erica Salcedo, Illustrator (Bright Light)
- *The Great Big Body Book* by Mary Hoffman; Ros Asquith, Illustrator (Frances Lincoln Children's Books)
- *We Toot: A Feminist Fable About Farting* by Ashley Wheelock and Arwen Evans; Sandie Sonke, Illustrator (House of Tomorrow)

BOUNDARIES AND CONSENT

- *Everyone's Got a Bottom* by Tess Rowley; Jodi Edwards, Illustrator (Family Planning Queensland)
- *Good Pictures, Bad Pictures Jr.: A Simple Plan to Protect Young Minds* by Kristen A. Jenson; Debbie Fox, Illustrator (Glen Cove Press)
- *Uncle Willy's Tickles: A Child's Right to Say No* (2nd ed.) by Marcie Aboff; Kathleen Gartner, Illustrator (Magination Press)
- *What Lily Knows* by Jessica Smarr (UN|HUSHED)

FAMILIES

- *A Family Is a Family Is a Family* by Sara O'Leary; Qin Leng, Illustrator (Groundwood Books/House of Anansi Press)
- *The Great Big Book of Families* by Mary Hoffman; Ros Asquith, Illustrator (Dial Books for Young Readers)

FEELINGS

- *Empathy Is Your Super Power: A Book About Understanding the Feelings of Others* by Cori Bussolari; Zach Grzeszkowiak, Illustrator (Rockridge Press)

- *Listening to My Body: A Guide to Helping Kids Understand the Connection Between Their Sensations (What the Heck Are Those?) and Feelings So That They Can Get Better at Figuring Out What They Need* (2nd ed.) by Gabi Garcia; Ying Hui Tan, Illustrator (Skinned Knee Publishing)
- *We Listen to Our Bodies* by Lydia Bowers; Isabel Muñoz, Illustrator (Free Spirit Publishing)

GENDER

- *A House for Everyone: A Story to Help Children Learn About Gender Identity and Gender Expression* by Jo Hirst; Naomi Bardoff, Illustrator (Jessica Kingsley Publishers)
- *It Feels Good to Be Yourself: A Book About Gender Identity* by Theresa Thorn; Noah Grigni, Illustrator (Henry Holt and Company)
- *Sparkle Boy* by Lesléa Newman; Maria Mola, Illustrator (Lee & Low Books)
- *Who Are You? The Kid's Guide to Gender Identity* by Brook Pessin-Whedbee; Naomi Bardoff, Illustrator (Jessica Kingsley Publishers)

REPRODUCTION

In addition to the books listed here, there are those available about specific reproduction topics, including adoption, egg and embryo donation, foster families, sperm donation, and surrogacy.

- *Nine Months: Before a Baby Is Born* by Miranda Paul; Jason Chin, Illustrator (Holiday House)
- *The Science of Babies: A Little Book for Big Questions About Bodies, Birth and Families* by Deborah Roffman; Frank Cable, Illustrator (Birdhouse Kids Media)

- *Where Did I Come From? The Facts of Life Without Any Nonsense and With Illustrations* (50th anniversary ed.) by Peter Mayle; Arthur Robins, Illustrator (Citadel Press)

SEXUALITY, ALL TOPICS

- *It's Not the Stork! A Book About Girls, Boys, Babies, Bodies, Families, and Friends* by Robie H. Harris; Michael Emberley, Illustrator (Candlewick Press)

Other Resources

- Clementine Wants to Know! app to use together with your child the first few times: Available for download from your online app store
- UN|HUSHED Living Things: A Reproduction Activity card deck: https://unhushed.org

Chapter 9

In the Moment:

Responding to Surprising Questions and Situations

If you've gotten shocking questions from your child, congratulations! That means your child is curious about the world and feels comfortable asking you about it. Whether it's a surprising question or an unforeseen situation, it's helpful to be prepared. Having a plan ahead of time helps us stay calm and think of the most appropriate way to respond. Even to a parent who is knowledgeable and comfortable with topics of sexuality, some questions can feel like a snowball in the face when we're least expecting it. In response, your mind may freeze in shock, or the questions may start to flow: "Why is she asking that?!" "What should I say?" Here, we give you a framework for a way you can answer surprising questions.

WHEN YOU ENCOUNTER SURPRISING QUESTIONS

In the moment when you encounter a surprising question, you may not be able to run away, search for this book, and cast about for a dog-eared page with the four steps you are supposed to use. We don't expect you to do that. Hopefully, however, the ideas provided with each step will sink in, and you'll get used to using them over time. The four steps we suggest for deer-in-the-headlights questions are *pause*, *validate*, *clarify*, and *answer*.

1. Pause

When you encounter a question that takes you off guard, the first thing you can do is this: Pause. Take a deep breath. Don't say anything for a few seconds. Remind yourself that what you want in the long run is to be an askable parent. You want your child to continue to come to *you* when they have questions about sexuality.

So, before you respond to your child, ask yourself, "Am I opening the door to future conversations, or am I shutting it?" Then use these next steps to answering questions: validate, clarify, and answer honestly.

2. Validate, Validate, Validate!

You want your child to know they can always ask you questions about sexuality. Reward their questions by telling them you are glad they asked. (Also, this gives you a little more time to breathe and think if you need it.)

 What you can say:
- "That's a great question."
- "I'm glad you asked that."
- "It's really cool that you're thinking about that."
- "I love what a curious kid you are."

3. Clarify

What exactly is being asked? What does your child already know? By understanding the question more completely, you will avoid giving irrelevant or confusing information.

208

What you can say:

- "What have you heard about that already?"
- "Why do you ask?"
- "Where did you hear that word/about that?"

4. Answer in Stages, Encourage Discussion

In the sections that follow, we offer examples of questions young children might ask and give suggestions for language you could use to answer their questions. If the question is values based, share your family's beliefs. You can also invite discussion and acknowledge family and community value differences.

WHAT YOU CAN SAY TO TODDLERS

For most toddler questions, you can give brief, simple answers. Wait for follow-up questions, rather than explaining everything at once. How simple you keep it will depend on the age and personality of the child and what you've told them already. You know your child best.

Question:	**What you can say:**
"Is that a man or a woman?"	"I'm not sure how they identify themselves. Some people don't think of themselves as either a woman or a man. Others can feel that they are both."
	"I'm not sure how they think of themselves. But they seem to be dressing very feminine, like a woman (or very masculine, like a man, or in a way that is neither feminine nor masculine)."

(continues)

209

(*continued*)

Question:	What you can say:
"How did the baby get in there?"	"Babies are created when an egg from one person gets together with a sperm from another person. The egg and sperm combine together and then grow into a baby in a part of the body called the uterus."
"How did the baby get out?"	"Babies usually get squeezed out through the vagina. The vagina is a stretchy tube that goes out from the uterus, where the baby grows."
"What is that (*pointing to a tampon or menstrual pad*)?"	"It's called a tampon (or menstrual pad). It's used when a person has what is called a *period*. When a person has a period, blood comes out of the vagina, and this is used to soak up the blood. They are not hurt; it's a natural thing that happens."
"Why can't I come into the bathroom?"	"Because sometimes people want privacy in the bathroom."
"Where's your penis?"	"I don't have a penis or scrotum. I have a vulva and vagina. Some people have a penis and scrotum, others have a vulva and vagina, and a few people have a different collection of parts."
"Why do you have hair there (*pointing to genitals*)?"	"Adults have hair on their genitals. When you change from being a child to an adult, you will get hair on your genitals too."
"Will you touch me here (*pointing to genitals*)?"	"Your genitals are special, and only you get to touch them unless I'm helping you with something like cleaning off poop or if your genitals are hurting."
"Why is your butt so jiggly?"	"Different people's bodies are different. Some people have a softer, squishier butt, and others do not."

WHAT YOU CAN SAY TO KINDERGARTNERS

Many of the questions and answers in the preceding toddler examples are still relevant for kindergartners. However, the questions kindergartners ask may also be more complex, and 5- and 6-year-olds are able to understand longer and more complex answers. How complex you make your answers will depend on the age and personality of the child and what you've told them already. You know your child best.

Question:	**What you can say:**
"How does the sperm get to the egg?"	"There are different ways that an egg and sperm can get together. You know how eggs come from a person with a vagina, uterus, and ovaries, and sperm comes from a person with a penis, scrotum, and testicles? Well, one of the most common ways a baby is made is when a penis and vagina fit together. Two people can decide they want to do that together because it feels good. Then, if an egg is traveling from the ovaries, and sperm travel from the testicles, the egg and sperm can meet up. Does that make sense?" "There are also other ways an egg and sperm can get together. Do you want to talk about those?"
"Today, I kissed Julia [classmate] the way you kiss mommy because I love her, but the teacher got really upset and told me to never do that again. What did I do wrong?"	"Wow, that must have been hard for you when your teacher got so upset. It's true that when people love each other, they sometimes like to kiss, and I can understand why you would do that. *But* that kind of kissing is something we do only with family. Hugs and cuddles you can do with your friends. Even though you did something that we only do with family, I wish your teacher didn't get so upset about it. It was an honest mistake, and I understand why you did it."

(continues)

(continued)

Question:	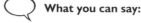 What you can say:
"Alex has two daddies. Can I have two daddies too?"	"Having two daddies sounds very special! Who else is in Alex's family? Let's think about who is in your family, starting with: Who are your parents? Who else loves you and takes care of you?"
"Why do dogs hump people's legs?"	"You know how people's genitals are really sensitive, and it can feel good to touch them? Dogs' genitals are the same way, and they are usually humping because it feels good to them."
"When will I get my breasts?"	"Breasts are something that grown-ups have. When your body changes from being a kid body to an adult body, that's called *puberty*. During puberty, kids with a vulva typically get breasts. Kids with a penis also sometimes get swelling of that area when they go through puberty, but then it goes away. People go through puberty at different ages. Usually, it starts at about age 11 or 12, but it can also start earlier or later."
"Why do people put naked videos online?"	"When people go through puberty, they often start to have sexual desires—feelings about themselves or toward other people. Some people enjoy seeing other people naked or being sexual with each other. It's not a bad thing for an adult to do, but there can be problems with putting pictures and videos online. For instance, usually the videos online are not realistic. They often don't show how people look or behave in real life, but some people start to think that's how sexual relationships should really be." "There are other problems, too, like sometimes the people in the videos aren't very nice to each other. Because it's made for adults, it's not good for kids to watch. Once you are older and you already have experiences in the real world, then you can decide for yourself if it's good for you."

WHEN YOU CAN'T ANSWER THEIR QUESTION

Many of the questions young children ask are simple enough that we can answer them in a quick and straightforward manner. There may be times when you need to delay a response to a child's question. Still, kids always deserve an answer, even if it's at a later time. One reason you may delay answering is that you may not know the answer. Similarly, you may really want to take time to think about how you want to answer their question. At other times, you may be in a situation in which the discussion you want to have isn't convenient or appropriate. In cases like this, make sure to validate their question first. Then acknowledge that you don't have an answer right now or that it's not a good time to talk about it. You can tell your child that you will find out the answer or that you need to think about it more. Make sure to follow up.

Follow-up is critically important. Your child probably won't forget that they've asked the question. When you come back to them later with an answer, you've validated their question and their trust in you. In addition, not providing an answer can prompt children to inquire elsewhere. Answers from other adults or children may not provide correct information or the messages you want them to hear.

WHEN YOU'RE TOO UNCOMFORTABLE
TO ANSWER THEIR QUESTION

Some of the questions children ask may make us uncomfortable. If you get really flustered, you can validate their questions and acknowledge your feelings at the same time.

 What you can say:

"It's funny. Talking about that makes me feel a little awkward. I really want to talk about it with you, though. Isn't it funny how some things can be weird to talk about sometimes?"

Allegra
BROOKLYN PARK, MINNESOTA

Mother to two children
Age when first child was born: 29

Ugh, I hate traffic! We really do only have two seasons here: winter and road construction, and today was a doozy! It took me 90 minutes to drive 11 miles this morning, and on the way home, with Violet in the car seat, the 45-minute drive felt more like 45 years. (Seriously, they need some kind of tubing system for potty-trained toddlers when they are in the car. "Mommy, I have to pee!" becomes a four-letter word when you are in bumper to bumper!)

Anyway, traffic is really not the point of this story. The point is this: I had heard stories from other parents who had been tongue-tied when facing some awkward situation with their kid, but I hadn't yet experienced this in my own parenthood journey—until today!

As we were racing down the freeway at a speed of 0 miles per hour, Violet was looking out the window, eating crackers and singing to herself. Suddenly, from the back seat, comes her dear little voice: "Mommy, what is a lover?" I pause and ask her, "What did you say, sweetie?" And again she says, "Mommy, what is a lover?" I realize that the reason we are stopped is because there is a stalled vehicle a bit ahead of me, and personnel have arrived on the scene to help us navigate through this challenge. (Where are the personnel in this car to help me navigate this challenge?!)

As I am steering my way gingerly around other cars, I mumble something along the lines of "there are lots of different kinds of people in the world, and sometimes people fall in love with each other, the way your mommy and daddy are, and they want to show each other how much they care, and. . . ." Thankfully, I didn't have to get too much further than that because trying to explain a romantic partner in age-appropriate ways to a 3-year-old was making me want to rear-end the car in front of me as a distraction.

Fortunately, I didn't have to elaborate because Violet said, "Mommy, you aren't making sense. I was trying to use the potty today, and our teacher kept telling all of us that when we were done to push the lover. I don't know what a lover is. I just wanted to flush the toilet!" Ah, yes, me describing a LOVER when you are trying to understand a LEVER is not super helpful, is it, my child? This parenting stuff is tough. I need a nap. Is it appropriate to nap an hour before my bedtime?

WHEN YOU ENCOUNTER SURPRISING SITUATIONS

Surprising situations, like surprising questions, can take us off guard. These situations vary and can include behaviors, such as asking to see or touch other people's genitals or breasts or touching their own genitals or nipples. These are developmentally expected behaviors, and, at the same time, we want to help our child establish healthy boundaries. Here we provide five ideas for how you could respond. In short, the steps are pause, validate, satiate curiosity, keep the conversation going, and talk with other parents.

1. Pause: Mitigate Embarrassment or Shame

Like surprising questions, when we are taken by surprise, it can be helpful to take a moment to let the flush in our face settle down. Take a slow, deep breath. Notice how you're feeling in your body.

One way we can help kids not to feel embarrassment or shame over a situation is by regulating our own feelings and responding in a positive way. If the behavior you encounter is really concerning to you, you can still keep calm in the moment. Staying calm will help your child, regardless of the situation you have discovered. Later on, you can take time to think about what happened, make a game plan, and address the concerning behavior.

215

2. Validate: Let Them Know Curiosity Is Normal and Boundaries Are a Must

Remember that young children are exploring everything, including bodies, and haven't yet learned about all the boundaries we think are important. Furthermore, much of the way they explore is through touch and experimentation.

After you pause and take a moment to collect yourself, focus on emphasizing that curiosity is normal and good. Then you can remind your child about appropriate boundaries.

 What you can say:

- "I see you're really curious about genitals. They are definitely very interesting! And, genitals are something we keep private."
- "Hey, kids, I know bodies are super cool, but your genitals are just for you."

3. Satiate Curiosity

Give kids a safe and appropriate way to satisfy their curiosity. We like curiosity!

 What you can say:

- "We have a lot of books that show genitals. Later today, we will look at them."
- "Here are some books and toys that are all about bodies. Why don't we look at them together?"

4. Keep the Conversation Going

By keeping your tone positive and satiating curiosity, you are keeping the door open for future discussion. In addition, the work you do every day by making small comments about sexuality, reading books together on the subject, and answering questions when they arise, all communicate to your child that they can go to you with questions or thoughts. That said, you can always explicitly tell them that they can come to you with any questions or thoughts they have.

5. Talk With the Parents of Any Other Children Involved

Any time boundaries are crossed with a child who isn't your own, it's important to inform the caregiver of that other child. If other parents aren't informed about what is developmentally normal, you can suggest some of the parent resources we have recommended. Hopefully, the other parent will be grateful that you handled the situation appropriately.

A True Story

Let's use an example of a true story to explore how we might respond:

> A 6-year-old girl had another child her age over for a playdate. While checking on the children, who were playing in the girl's bedroom, the mom discovered them engaging in "you show me yours, and I'll show you mine." The mom understood normal curiosity about genitals. What really concerned her was that the children were taking pictures of their genitals with an iPad that the child usually used for games and videos.

We can imagine the feeling this mom must have had when she discovered this scene. Is what happened here the result of normal curiosity? Or should she be concerned about the photographs? Why did they have the idea to take pictures? Was it because they took pictures of everything, and they were being silly? Or is it because one of them has experienced child sexual abuse and is acting that out? *As an exercise, before you read on, think about what you would have done.*

Here is an idea for how we—Laura and Karen—would handle the situation using the aforementioned steps: pause, validate, satiate curiosity, keep the conversation going, and talk with other parents:

- Pause: Take a deep breath, and remind ourselves that this is not an emergency. Take another deep breath to think about what to say.
- Validate and satiate curiosity: Say something like, "Hey, kiddos, our genitals are private. So, let's only be naked around (our family, mom and dad, and sometimes doctors—choose your version). Bodies *are* really cool, though! We have some great books about bodies and genitals, and we could lend one to you (friend) if your parent is okay with that. Why don't we all get a snack together and think of another activity to play?"
- Keep the conversation going: Later on, when we are in a calm, connected place with our own child, like snuggled up and getting ready to read a bedtime story or riding together in the car, we have a conversation about what happened.
  - We say something like, "I noticed when you were playing with your friend that you were taking pictures of your genitals. Have you ever done that before? It's okay if you have. I won't be mad. It's just important that I know." We explain that when we take pictures, whatever is in the picture isn't really private anymore because other people can see it. Because genitals are private, we shouldn't show them to people or take pictures of them.
  - And we conclude by saying, "If you're ever curious about bodies and genitals, you can ask me, you can use a mirror to look at your own genitals, or we have a lot of books about

them." (If you want more information about child sexual abuse specifically, refer to Chapter 5.)

- Talk with other parents: Because another child was involved, we want to talk with the playdate's parent(s) in private about what happened. We offer them the use of an age-appropriate book if they don't have one for their child and suggest they check in with their child about whether they've been exposed to pictures of genitals.
  - Talking with another child's parents about these things can be really uncomfortable, especially when other families don't have the same values around open discussion regarding sexual health. Still, it's best to be open with other parents about events that involve their child's sexuality.

BECOMING (MORE) UNSHOCKABLE

We want our kids to feel comfortable telling us about anything or asking any question they have. One of the most important ways to foster that comfort and confidence is to be unshockable. Realistically, we will be taken aback by some of the things kids do and say—and that's okay. We can, however, work on being less reactive.

Here are a few suggestions for starting that process. You can find a more comprehensive list in Chapter 2, which is all about self-awareness.

Contemplate Your Feelings and Reactions

Awareness of our own feelings around sexuality is an essential step to teaching our kids about healthy sexuality. We all have different responses to learning about and teaching about sexuality, and feelings of discomfort around this topic are common. If we are going to do a great job teaching young people about sexuality, however, we do need to get more comfortable with the ideas ourselves.

So, notice how you feel and perhaps take some time to think about why you feel that way. Do some of the exercises in Chapter 2. If you think about these things now, they won't take you so much by surprise when they come up with your child.

Practice, Practice, Practice

Help yourself become more used to these topics and terms. Once you have gotten some of the children's books we recommend, read through them by yourself. If you notice discomfort, read through them multiple times by yourself. Are there specific words that make you feel uncomfortable? Laura spoke with one mom who looked at herself in the mirror and said, "Vagina" 100 times to help herself feel more comfortable using the word with her daughter.

You can also practice responding to awkward or surprising situations. We provide an exercise for this purpose near the end of the chapter. You can also read through the true stories throughout this book and think about how you would respond. What would you say and do? Having some scripts ready that you can adjust to different situations will help you feel prepared in the moment.

Talk With Other Parents

Another way to practice is by talking with other parents. You will be amazed and amused by other families' stories of children learning about sexuality. By talking with other parents, you can get ideas for how to respond and start to imagine how you would react in similar situations. When we hear about the awkward and hilarious situations other parents have encountered, it makes it easier to discuss

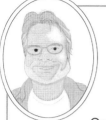

Will

EASTON, PENNSYLVANIA

Father to two children
Age when first child was born: 30

Once when Ryan was little, he had to tag along with Mom, Dad (me), and Grandpa (my father) to one of Mom's doctor's appointments. The gynecologist's office. A precocious reader, Ryan took in the headlines of one of the health magazines. From across the room, he called to his grandpa, "Papa, what's a period?" All eyes shifted like those of spectators at a tennis match to my father, who was squirming and unable to find a good answer other than: "Let's ask your grandmother later."

I wonder if I would have handled it any better. Even now, decades later, it's hard to imagine the words that would flow out easily, knowing that my response would be subject to the scrutiny (or entertainment) of everyone else in the room. My dad probably scored an A+ in terms of social expectations. Men are not supposed to know the answers to such questions, much less teach their grandsons! Had I been there and succeeded in giving an honest and accurate response, I suspect it would have been received with grimaces for violating expectations of social taboos.

Years later, I was interviewed by a men's magazine doing a story about fatherhood. They kept trying to steer me to reinforce the idea that it is difficult for men to talk to children about sex. Although I was mindful of my dad's experience and the continuous need to battle social expectations, I kept resisting their premise. Eventually, I yielded just a little bit and acknowledged that it's sometimes okay to have Mom answer a question if Dad feels uncomfortable. The magazine seized on this point and made it a focus of its article. We have so much work to do to shift the gender-based biases and assumptions while also making it more and more comfortable for dads to be the reliable sources of sexual information their children need them to be.

our own. The more we talk about it, the less awkward it becomes in real life.

EXERCISE: RESPONDING TO SURPRISING SITUATIONS

This is an exercise to give you some practice responding to surprising situations. For this exercise, you can use the help of a friend. If that feels uncomfortable for you, do the exercise yourself.

What follows are descriptions of situations that parents commonly face. Ask your friend to read them to you and then respond as though you were really responding to those situations. How would you behave? What would you say? Maybe you indeed have been in such a situation. What did you do?

Don't worry about having the right answer. Pay attention to how you feel when you respond. Do you feel confident and immediately have a response in mind? Do you freeze up and notice your mind go blank? Do you giggle, feel anxious, or feel like just skipping this one? After you respond to each prompt, your partner can ask you, "How did that feel?"

Another way you can approach this exercise is to do it with a coparent if you have one. You can take turns responding to the prompts and then discuss your responses.

Let's start:

- You walk into the playroom and see that your child has taken off their clothes and is exploring their genitals. You respond by . . .
- Your child comes home and says their friend has a "va-jay-jay" down there. You respond by . . .
- You and your child see a pregnant person, and your child asks, "How did the baby get in there?" You respond by . . .

- You find your child with their hand in their underwear while watching TV. You respond by . . .
- You find your child playing with another child of the same age, showing their genitals to each other. You respond by . . .
- Your son tells you that he wants to paint his nails and wear a skirt to school. Or, your daughter tells you she hates her long hair and wants to cut it short so it won't be in her way when she's playing football. You respond by . . .
- You are in the grocery store, and your child laughs and says very loudly, "My penis/vulva feels funny!" You respond by . . .
- Your child says, "What does *fuck* mean?" You respond by . . .

After you finish the exercise, you can consider the following questions together with your partner: What are other situations you've heard about or encountered? How do you want to respond to them if they were to arise now? How do your answers reflect your family values about sexuality? If you are coparenting, what are your partner's answers? Are you sending the same messages?

SUMMARY

- One of the keys to responding well to surprising questions is to pause before you act. Regardless of the situation, staying calm will help.
- Before you respond, ask yourself, "How can I keep the door open to future conversations?"
- No matter how surprised you may feel, try to stay positive. You can do this by praising your child's curiosity and recognizing that sexual behavior and curiosity are normal.
- Pausing and staying positive can be difficult to do in the moment. Practicing these skills in other situations, in your mind, or with

another adult (e.g., using role-play) can help you when you need to do it in the moment.

A RESOURCE FOR PARENTS

- *How to Talk So Little Kids Will Listen: A Survival Guide to Life With Children Ages 2–7* by Joanna Faber and Julie King; Coco Faber, Tracey Faber, and Sam Faber Manning, Illustrators (Scribner)

Chapter 10
What Comes Next?

Literally everything.

We don't mean to be sarcastic here, but it's true. Everything else that will come comes after what is in this book. Here are a few (although not all!) of the topics relating to sex, sexuality, human development, and parenting that will likely arise in the next 10 to 20 years. These are some (but not all) of the possible highlights (or lowlights, depending on your perspective):

- the connection between sexual intercourse and reproduction
- puberty
- first conversation about porn
- sex education classes
- first crush, first love
- first heartbreak
- first sex

We don't tell you these things to scare you or to overwhelm you. Indeed, we hope that, instead, you're excited by them! There is a lot to be excited about here: so many possibilities for connection, love, and pleasure and so many possibilities of learning, understanding, and humanity. Let's go over these possibilities and the ways you could actualize the best possible outcome for each of them.

THE CONNECTION BETWEEN SEXUAL INTERCOURSE
AND REPRODUCTION

This is often what parents mean when they ask us—Laura and Karen—"When should we have THE TALK with our child?" People learn the specifics of sexual intercourse and reproduction all across the lifespan. Some already know about it before they turn 5, and some are well into adulthood before they find out. However, it is generally better for people to learn these details when they're young—before or at the beginning of puberty. When they learn about it before this age, they incorporate it into their general understanding of the world that just exists, without judgment. We find that if children learn these details after this age, they can struggle with it and what it means about them, their origins, and their parents' sexuality.

Most parents have never had the experience of explaining intercourse to another person for the first time (at least until after their oldest child!). Figuring out how to do this can feel daunting. As we've mentioned, practicing with a coparent, therapist, or friend definitely helps. Here are five important points to include in that conversation:

1. For a pregnancy to start, an egg and a sperm come together. People with vulvas usually have something inside their abdomen called ovaries, where they have eggs. People with penises usually have something called testicles that hang below their penises and make sperm. (Tell your child what their body makes or is expected to make when they get older.)

2. Egg and sperm can come together in a few different ways. The most common way is for two people to decide together to put one person's penis into one person's vagina. Penises are usually erect (larger and harder) when they are put into a vagina.

3. Sperm come out of the penis and go up into the uterus and then into the fallopian tubes, where they wait.

4. Usually, one egg is released every month (it alternates which ovary it is released from). When the egg is released, if there are sperm in the fallopian tubes, one sperm may fertilize the egg.
5. The fertilized egg then goes back down the fallopian tubes and can implant into the uterus. This is when a pregnancy starts.

With complex topics like this, it is likely that the child will need to have it described several times, potentially over several years, before they fully grasp the details.

PUBERTY

The ways bodies change from those of children to those of adults is a complex process that takes years—and so do conversations about puberty! As your child grows beyond age 5 and toward ages 8, 9, and 10, conversations will turn from noticing physical differences between them (a child, currently) and you (an adult, currently) to the specifics of the physical changes that will grow their bodies from that of a child into that of an adult.

The most important topics to bring up before they happen are menstruation and penile ejaculation. Both of these experiences can be frightening for children who don't know to expect them in the course of puberty.

Other important topics to include in your conversations about puberty are these:

- Puberty starts at different times for different people. There is no "right" or "wrong" time to start or end puberty.
- Everyone experiences some parts of puberty, like growing hair in new places, growing taller, and their bodies making different smells.
- People experience some parts of puberty based on their bodies— like people with penises are more likely to have their voices

drop, and people with vaginas are more likely to develop larger breasts. It's important to know what kinds of changes different bodies will go through because it's important to be kind to everyone about these changes. They are not things that people chose.

FIRST CONVERSATION ABOUT PORN

The average age of first porn viewing is around 14. Most parents aren't ready to start talking with their kids about porn by that age. It's okay if you feel uncomfortable, but pornography still needs to become part of your conversation about sex and sexuality at some point in middle school. Even if your child hasn't seen pornography by then, their peers have.

The way to build up to this conversation over time is by starting to talk early on with your child about the media they are consuming. When your conversation about the representation of love and dating, and marriage and pregnancy, starts with animated children's movies, it will be easier to transition into conversations about sex and sexuality in nonporn media. This will eventually lead to openings to talk about media that actually show sexual activity or pornography.

All of the critical techniques that you will want to apply to conversations about nonporn media are similarly useful for talking about porn. Here are some questions to bring into those conversations:

- "Who made this?"
- "Why did they make it?"
- "How does it make you feel?"
- "How are they making you feel that way?"
- "Why are they making you feel that way?"

- "How do the actors or performers look like they feel?"
- "Do you think that's how most people would feel in that situation?"

With pornography, it's important to share with younger teenagers that pornography sex is not the same thing as real sex. Pornography sex is usually created with a very certain audience in mind and can be exploitative of the performers.

SEX EDUCATION CLASSES

At some point in your child's education, they will ideally have a series of sexuality education classes. As a parent, you'll be faced with a decision about what classes and when to enroll them—or to withhold enrollment—in a school environment.

Comprehensive sexuality education classes that take place outside of the family dynamic are very important as children grow out of puberty. This form of education helps kids understand that they aren't alone. It builds skill in talking with peers about consent and body image. It gives them another adult to help them sort through their questions (hopefully anonymously as well as in class). It also delays sexual activity and increases the likelihood of using condoms and other birth control. In short, comprehensive sexuality education reduces the risks that sex and sexuality pose for young people during their adolescent years. We highly recommend finding a way for your child to receive these classes during their early adolescent years (if not throughout the lifespan, which is even better!).

Some sex education classes are more harmful than beneficial, though. If you find a class that is not inclusive of a wide range of values and identities (both conservative and liberal), your child might be hurt by participating. However, a really good sex education class can offer immense benefit for your child and for your parent–child communication.

In addition to inclusivity, consider the facilitator training and experience, the values of the curriculum and the ways in which it engages participants (is it mostly focused on the facilitator expressing their point of view, or activity based, or something else?), and whether you (the parent) can view the materials. Ask how the curriculum fits into the scope and sequence of your child's school. And then, after a program has gotten started, ask your child how it's going. Let them know that you're interested in talking with them about sex ed. Even if they don't want to share much (which is fine!), you're making it clear that you are open to talking and you're aware of the content they're learning.

FIRST CRUSH, FIRST LOVE

The first time that a person feels a special kind of *zing* when they see or are around a certain person, it is often a powerful moment in their life. Whether this happens when they are 5 or 10 or 15 or 20 or even older, it is often a moment of awakening to a new element of themselves.

When children bring these feelings to you, it is a moment of trust and disclosure. When they don't bring these feelings to you, it is a moment of stepping into their own selves. Either way, when you are able to accept their disclosure choices as their own and support them in that moment, you work toward connection and parent–child trust.

FIRST HEARTBREAK

The first heartbreak can come immediately on the heels of a child's first crush or love, or it can be many years later. Either way, acknowledging the pain as real and valid is necessary and builds the connection between the two of you. This means that even if you don't really understand their sadness—whether because of their age or the length of the relationship or the other person's personality—understand that your child's feelings are real and true for them, at this time, and that's what matters most.

When you respond to your child's heartbreak by connecting with their expressed emotions, you're telling your child that you are a safe person to share their emotions with. You're telling them that you are on their team. When you respond to your child's heartbreak by teasing them or trying to talk them out of feeling sad, you're telling them that they can't share with you.

These lingering feelings of connection between you and your child are the most important elements of these conversations, rather than anything specific about dealing with heartbreak. They are what the child will remember most deeply when they need to talk with an adult about something painful or worrisome.

FIRST SEX

The first time a person has sex (whatever that means to them), there are so many cultural tropes and assumptions to navigate. Here are a few of them:

- The first time you have sex, if you are being penetrated, it will hurt, and you will possibly bleed.
- Virginity (not having had sex) is a measure of a person's (especially a girl's) value.
- You can't get pregnant or catch a sexually transmitted infection the first time you have sex.

None of these things is true. Helping your child feel authentically in charge of their own body, a process that includes knowing when cultural messages are inaccurate, will support your relationship and their developing sexuality. It provides them with accurate information on which to make safer, healthier decisions for themselves and their partners.

As a preteen grows into a teenager, having explicit family-based conversations about the elements involved in a sexual debut, along with other topics, allows you to share your family values, push back against cultural expectations, and build a relationship platform. Your child will come to rely on that relationship, knowing they can come and talk with you should they or one of their peers have sex and be in need of support.

TESTIMONIALS

We want to leave you here, at the end of the book, with testimonials of parents and children who went through these early years of life talking about sex and sexuality in positive, affirming ways. All of these children have grown into adulthood, so the thoughts that they and their parents share here are looking back on many years of growth and development.

As with all of the personal stories shared in this book, the names have been changed to maintain the privacy of the writers and their family members.

Family Unit 1

Izabella and Jason are parents to seven children, including Elena, Storm, and Stevie. The parents and these three children share their experiences.

Izabella, Age 45, White, Cisgender Woman

The topic of how to talk about sex struck me as one of the more clear-cut decisions of my parenting. When I was first a mother at age 23, I didn't have the knowledge base I needed, but over the next few years, I went on to be inspired to find answers and become a solid resource for them because I watched as friends struggled to deal with basic questions about bodies and pleasure. I didn't intend to center sexuality education, but in a way it became the centerpiece of their upbringing because being sex-positive formed a core value.

Over 20 years later, I see that as the value deepened, the concept of sex-positivity became the water we swam in. I tended to forget that other families didn't answer questions frankly until I found myself confronted with a visiting friend of the kids who were desperate for answers and helped out of their shame around sex and their bodies.

Sexuality became mundane, a topic that could be talked about openly, yet that didn't mean that the societal norms and negativity didn't seep in. The kids received those harsh narratives in differing ways according to the microcosms they created around themselves. Consistently addressing moralistic messaging hasn't even been enough to totally counterbalance the sex-negativity in their larger world. The primary motivator to continually educate my kids in a sex-positive way was reinspired daily as the world at large continued to demonize pleasure and make taboos out of normal behaviors.

Jason, Age 55, White, Gender-Fluid

There are so many clear positives of a household that approaches sexuality as "talkaboutable." These are the positive outcomes I experience as a parent. The kids have been able to explore their sexuality in the open, talking with us parents and each other about everything. I see them take opportunities to explore and question, and experiment with presentation and identity. This makes it easier for them to discover for themselves what fits them and what doesn't, and to create their own place in the world instead of picking from the predefined menu of choices provided by the larger culture.

233

They've had access to enough medically accurate sexual health information to make informed choices about health care (immunizations and safer sex practices) and to advocate for themselves in sexual situations they might find themselves in. They're aware of the value of and need for consent, which means they are safer in relationships themselves and are safer people to be in a relationship with. So, as a parent, I get a lot of peace of mind knowing that they are going to be able to navigate the sexual aspect of their own growth consciously and with intention.

Elena, Age 22, White, Cisgender Woman

There are no expectations in my family's house when it comes to sex, relationships, or self-identity. I have a lack of guilt and know that for every or any question I may have, there is an answer. I know that so long as I am safe, happy, and causing no harm, all requirements are met. This is a privilege that few people grow up with that I am grateful to have experienced.

Storm, Age 20, White, Cisgender Man

One of the positives of growing up in a family that discussed sexuality and sexual orientation openly is that none of us have ever had to "come out" as a sexual orientation other than straight. That's not to say that all of us are straight, just that we feel comfortable being who we are. There was no need to distinguish ourselves as different or abnormal because we grew up with a normalized view of sexuality and sexual orientations.

Stevie, Age 18, White, Cisgender Woman

No matter what kind of situation I am in—when I need help or need to ask a question—I can always find a way to get it. I don't have to look it up.

Family Unit 2

Patty, age 55, is a White, cisgender woman and a mom to three children. This is her story.

The best part of talking to your children openly and honestly about sexuality in their life is it sets the stage for your conversations when they are teenagers and adults. Before they were 5, I taught my children the correct names of the parts of their bodies, about privacy, where babies come from, and that all families are special. My children learned I was an askable parent and that nothing was off limits for us to discuss.

When they were approaching puberty, we had easy, relaxed conversations about how their bodies were changing. They came to me to talk when they first fell in love. My youngest was able to come out to us their sophomore year in high school because they knew we would be happy whoever they were. We talk about their primary relationships. Like love and faith, sexuality has been part of their lives and our conversations since the beginning.

Family Unit 3

Mary, age 73, is a White, cisgender woman and a mom to two adult children. This is her story.

I was raised by forward-thinking, respectful parents who were more European in perspective than American. My papa immigrated from Italy at 14; my mama was the eighth child of 11 born to Italian immigrant parents; she was the fourth born in America. Culturally, my parents were warm, open, deeply committed to family (*la mia famiglia*) and determined to raise me American. I was not taught Italian (although they seldom cursed in English, so I can swear like a sailor in Italian).

My mama prepared me for my period, and that was the first formal conversation we had about sexuality. Informally, however, they were ahead of their time, at least in America. I was taught correct names for body parts and given messages about consent and healthy relationships in both words and example. They were married 64 years before they died 4 months apart; their life was one long model of what a healthy relationship could be.

Papa was unique among the fathers of my friends. For example, when I started my period, my mama told me I could no longer jump rope with my friends because "I was a woman" now. I was 10; it was 1960. Papa took me aside and told me I was still me—a better me with the capability of becoming a mother someday. I was raised Catholic, so the idea that I might choose to be childless didn't even cross their minds!

It was Papa who dripped self-worth into me daily. If I had a new outfit, he would ask me to spin and then pronounce me the most beautiful daughter in the world. He said goodnight to me in Italian: "Buona note all figlia piu bella del mondo" ["Goodnight to the most beautiful daughter in the world"].

When I first went to Penn State to visit my future husband for the weekend, Papa walked me to the car. He asked, gently and with respect, if my future husband and I would have sex. We had not, as of yet. I remember I was not embarrassed. Papa was chaste and set wonderful boundaries, but he never stopped hugging me like some fathers when puberty began. He was open about sexuality in a casual, respectful, matter-of-fact way.

Again, remember the Catholicism. I was certain he would admonish me to be abstinent, but I could not lie to him. I told him we'd talked about it, and we weren't sure we were ready, so I thought not. He shrugged and asked me if we were preparing, just in case. We talked about protection, then I assured him we were considering the possibility very seriously. Papa smiled. "It will be hard," he said. I reassured him of our ability to decide and wait if we thought that was the right choice. His eyes twinkled. "No," he smiled, "I mean he will be hard."

I remember laughing and loving my papa so much. How often does a girl grow up in an atmosphere where the first man to love her does so with such incredible gentleness, consistency, and kindness?

My husband and I raised three children, who are now adults. I taught sexuality from 1981, and our first was born in 1976. From the start, I modeled my parents. Body parts were labeled correctly and taught with respect. Consent was taught from toddlerhood. I started teaching classes on growing up when our eldest was 9, mostly because I couldn't find a class that was open, body-positive, and affirming.

Generational trauma is real. Generational joy and openness and education and positive role-modeling in sexual health are also real. I was blessed to be part of a life-affirming cycle, where bodies were amazing and sexuality was beautiful.

IT'S WORTH IT TO DO THE HARD WORK

As Mary said, generational trauma is real. It takes courage and effort to stop an intergenerational cycle of trauma, ignorance, or shame around sexuality. Doing the work to heal yourself while simultaneously teaching your child about healthy sexuality can be difficult and uncomfortable, but it is also rewarding. You can create a new cycle of learning about sexuality and be a better role model. You can create a family in which there is open communication; stronger relationships; and happier, healthier futures for the next generation.

SUMMARY

- As younger children grow into older children and then teenagers, their understanding of sexuality (both in themselves and between themselves and other people) expands. Likewise, the kinds of conversations that they need expand dramatically. They will need to have a concrete understanding of human bodies and reproduction, the act of sex, puberty, pornography, crushes, heartbreak, sex education, and first-time intercourse. These are really just the very beginning conversations—and from here, they grow into so many more beautiful things and ways to connect.

• Know that when parents lay the groundwork for having forthright and open conversations about sex and sexuality during these early years, it pays off immensely by creating a lifelong conversation. The protective and connecting factors are so important.

RESOURCES FOR PARENTS

Today, there are a plethora of resources that support parents in their effort to help children develop healthy sexuality. We have provided many of our favorites here. As you look for resources on your own, we recommend double-checking that the materials are fact-, rather than opinion-, based.

Online

• *Amy Lang's Birds & Bees & Kids*: https://birdsandbeesand-kids.com/amy-lang-sex-education-expert
• *Every Body Curious* show on YouTube, which you can watch with your 9- to 12-year-old: https://www.youtube.com/playlist?list=PLFrqObEvDOwkfkcik9TOYgBh4RlhIXj-_
• *For Parents*, Planned Parenthood: https://www.plannedparenthood.org/learn/parents
• Sex Ed Rescue: https://sexedrescue.com
• Sex Positive Families: https://sexpositivefamilies.com
• *Six Minute Sex Ed* podcast; choose which age group is right for you, and listen with the family: Find via your favorite podcast application

Books

- *Beyond the Birds and the Bees: Bringing Home a New Message to Our Kids About Sex, Love, and Equality* by Bonnie J. Rough (Seal Press)
- *Breaking the Hush Factor: Ten Rules for Talking With Teenagers About Sex* by Karen Rayne (Impetus Books)
- *Talking to Your Kids About Sex: Turning "the Talk" Into a Conversation for Life* by Laura Berman (DK)

RESOURCES FOR KIDS

These are some of the resources we like for young people from kindergarten age through their teenage years. It's a good idea to research other resources in addition to these as your child grows. New books and new knowledge about sexuality are always becoming available. As children get older, they will begin to use books and other resources on their own, with less parental involvement. Still, reading the books they are reading (on your own) or visiting the same resources will help you to know what language, topics, and information they are learning about.

For Younger Children

- *It's Not the Stork! A Book About Girls, Boys, Babies, Bodies, Families, and Friends* by Robie H. Harris; Michael Emberley, Illustrator (Candlewick Press)
- *It's So Amazing: A Book About Eggs, Sperm, Birth, Babies, and Families* by Robie H. Harris; Michael Emberley, Illustrator (Candlewick Press)
- *Sex Is a Funny Word: A Book About Bodies, Feelings, and YOU* by Cory Silverberg and Fiona Smyth (Seven Stories Press)
- *Tell Me About Sex, Grandma* by Anastasia Higginbotham (Dottir Press)

For Preteens

If they are not already, your preteen will soon be able to access information about sexuality on their own. This is the time to make sure they know how to distinguish between healthy and unhealthy sources of information. You can start by providing some of the resources we have listed here, but also make sure to discuss media literacy and, specifically, how to parse out fact from fiction when searching online.

ONLINE

- AMAZE: https://amaze.org

BOOKS

- *It's Perfectly Normal: Changing Bodies, Growing Up, Sex, Gender, and Sexual Health* by Robie H. Harris; Michael Emberley, Illustrator (Candlewick Press)
- *Wait, What? A Comic Book Guide to Relationships, Bodies, and Growing Up* by Heather Corinna and Isabella Rotman; colored by Luke B. Howard (Limerence Press)
- *You Know, Sex: A Book About Bodies, Gender, Puberty, and Other Things* by Cory Silverberg and Fiona Smyth (Seven Stories Press)

For Teenagers

Teenagers find information and form opinions on their own. (Hopefully, they like to discuss those opinions with you!) Like preteens, they need to know about media literacy and how to distinguish between healthy and unhealthy sources of information. Here are resources you can provide to give examples of healthy, evidence-based sources of information.

ONLINE

- Scarleteen: https://www.scarleteen.com

BOOKS

- *GIRL: Love, Sex, Romance, and Being You* by Karen Rayne (Magination Press)
- *S.E.X.: The All-You-Need-to-Know Sexuality Guide to Get You Through Your Teens and Twenties* (2nd ed.) by Heather Corinna (Da Capo Lifelong Books)
- *Trans+: Love, Sex, Romance, and Being You* by Kathryn Gonzales and Karen Rayne (Magination Press)

REFERENCES

Allen, K. R., Gary, E. A., Lavender-Stott, E. S., & Kaestle, C. E. (2018). "I walked in on them": Young adults' childhood perceptions of sex and nudity in family and public contexts. *Journal of Family Issues*, *39*(15), 3804–3831. https://doi.org/10.1177/0192513X18793923

Aron, E. N. (2002). *The highly sensitive child: Helping our children thrive when the world overwhelms them*. Broadway Books.

Bekos, D., & Russo, T. (2017). The joyfully sexual infant in the room: A response to Frances Thomson-Salo and Campbell Paul. *Psychoanalytic Dialogues*, *27*(3), 338–343. https://doi.org/10.1080/10481885.2017.1308212

Bem, S. L. (1983). Gender schema theory and its implications for child development: Raising gender-aschematic children in a gender-schematic society. *Signs*, *8*, 598–616. https://doi.org/10.1086/493998

Bernier, J. (2014). *Straight talk about child sexual abuse: A prevention guide for parents*. Enough Abuse Campaign. https://www.enoughabuse.org/images/stories/Bookshelf/Straight_Talk/straighttalk_gba_interactiveREV.pdf

Breuner, C. C., Mattson, G., Committee on Adolescence, Committee on Psychosocial Aspects of Child and Family Health, Breuner, C. C., Adelman, W. P., Alderman, E. M., Garofalo, R., Marcell, A. V., Powers, M. E., Mph, M., Upadhya, K. K., Yogman, M. W., Bauer, N. S., Gambon, T. B., Lavin, A., Lemmon, K. M., Mattson, G., Rafferty, J. R., & Wissow, L. S. (2016). Sexuality education for children and adolescents. *Pediatrics*, *138*(2), Article e20161348. https://doi.org/10.1542/peds.2016-1348

Bukowski, W. M., Panarello, B., & Santo, J. B. (2017). Androgyny in liking and in being liked are antecedent to well-being in pre-adolescent boys and girls. *Sex Roles, 76*(11–12), 719–730. https://doi.org/10.1007/s11199-016-0638-6

Buss, A. H., Iscoe, I., & Buss, E. H. (1979). The development of embarrassment. *Journal of Psychology, 103*(2), 227–230.

Cacciatore, R. S. M., Ingman-Friberg, S. M.-L., Lainiala, L. P., & Apter, D. L. (2020). Verbal and behavioral expressions of child sexuality among 1–6-year-olds as observed by daycare professionals in Finland. *Archives of Sexual Behavior, 49*(7), 2725–2734. https://doi.org/10.1007/s10508-020-01694-y

Carter, C. (2021). Navigating young children's friendship selection: Implications for practice. *International Journal of Early Years Education.* Advance online publication. https://doi.org/10.1080/09669760.2021.1892600

Chung, Y., & Huang, H.-H. (2021). Cognitive-based interventions break gender stereotypes in kindergarten children. *International Journal of Environmental Research and Public Health, 18*(24), Article 13052. https://doi.org/10.3390/ijerph182413052

Council on Communications and Media, Hill, D., Ameenuddin, N., Reid Chassiakos, Y. L., Cross, C., Hutchinson, J., Levine, A., Boyd, R., Mendelson, R., Moreno, M., & Swanson, W. S. (2016). Media and young minds. *Pediatrics, 138*(5), Article e20162591. https://doi.org/10.1542/peds.2016-2591

Daly, A., & O'Sullivan, C. (2020). Sexuality education and international standards: Insisting upon children's rights. *Human Rights Quarterly, 42*(4), 835–858. https://doi.org/10.1353/hrq.2020.0043

Domek, G. J., Szafran, L. H., Bonnell, L. N., Berman, S., & Camp, B. W. (2020). Using finger puppets in the primary care setting to support caregivers talking with their infants: A feasibility pilot study. *Clinical Pediatrics, 59*(4–5), 380–387. https://doi.org/10.1177/0009922820903407

EL Education. (n.d.). *Characteristics of primary learners.* https://eleducation.org/resources/characteristics-of-primary-learners

Elia, J. P. (2009). School-based sexuality education: A century of sexual and social control. In E. Schroder & J. Kuriansky (Eds.), *Sexuality education: Past, present, and future: Vol. 1. History and information* (pp. 33–57). Praeger Publishers.

Halim, M. L. D., Walsh, A. S., Tamis-LeMonda, C. S., Zosuls, K. M., & Ruble, D. N. (2018). The roles of self-socialization and parent socialization in toddlers' gender-typed appearance. *Archives of Sexual Behavior*, 47(8), 2277–2285. https://doi.org/10.1007/s10508-018-1263-y

Ichikawa, H., & Yamaguchi, M. K. (2014). Infants' recognition of subtle facial expression. *Japanese Psychological Research*, 56(1), 15–23. https://doi.org/10.1111/jpr.12025

Katz-Wise, S. L., Galman, S. C., & Kidd, K. M. (2022). Parent/caregiver narratives of challenges related to raising transgender and/or nonbinary youth. *Journal of Family Issues*, 43(12), 3321–3345. https://doi.org/10.1177/0192513X211044484

Katz-Wise, S. L., Rosario, M., & Tsappis, M. (2016). Lesbian, gay, bisexual, and transgender youth and family acceptance. *Pediatric Clinics of North America*, 63(6), 1011–1025. https://doi.org/10.1016/j.pcl.2016.07.005

Kellogg, J. H. (1882). *Plain facts for old and young*. Segner.

Kinsey, A., Pomeroy, W., & Martin, C. (1948). *Sexual behavior in the human male*. Saunders.

Klika, J. B., & Conte, J. R. (Eds.). (2017). *The APSAC handbook on child maltreatment* (4th ed.). SAGE Publications.

Liberman, Z., Woodward, A. L., & Kinzler, K. D. (2017). Preverbal infants infer third-party social relationships based on language. *Cognitive Science*, 41(S3), 622–634. https://doi.org/10.1111/cogs.12403

Lovenheim, P. (2018). *The attachment effect: Exploring the powerful ways our earliest bond shapes our relationships and lives*. TarcherPerigee.

Mahler, M. S., Pine, F., & Bergman, A. (2018). *The psychological birth of the human infant: Symbiosis and individuation*. Routledge.

Marshall, N., & Shibazaki, K. (2020). Gender associations and musical instruments: Understanding the responses of nursery-aged children. *Educational Research*, 62(4), 455–473. https://doi.org/10.1080/00131881.2020.1836988

Martinello, E. (2020). Applying the ecological systems theory to better understand and prevent child sexual abuse. *Sexuality & Culture*, 24(1), 326–344. https://doi.org/10.1007/s12119-019-09629-z

Martino, S. C., Elliott, M. N., Corona, R., Kanouse, D. E., & Schuster, M. A. (2008). Beyond the "big talk": The roles of breadth and repetition in parent–adolescent communication about sexual topics. *Pediatrics*, 121(3), e612–e618. https://doi.org/10.1542/peds.2007-2156

May, L., Byers-Heinlein, K., Gervain, J., & Werker, J. F. (2011). Language and the newborn brain: Does prenatal language experience shape the neonate neural response to speech? *Frontiers in Psychology, 2*, Article 222. https://doi.org/10.3389/fpsyg.2011.00222

Mendelson, T., & Letourneau, E. J. (2015). Parent-focused prevention of child sexual abuse. *Prevention Science, 16*(6), 844–852. https://doi.org/10.1007/s11121-015-0553-z

Newton, E. K., Thompson, R. A., & Goodman, M. (2016). Individual differences in toddlers' prosociality: Experiences in early relationships explain variability in prosocial Behavior. *Child Development, 87*(6), 1715–1726. https://doi.org/10.1111/cdev.12631

Nobre, J. N. P., Prat, B. V., Santos, J. N., Santos, L. R., Pereira, L., da C. Guedes, S., Ribeiro, R. F., & de S. Morales, R. L. (2020). Qualidade de uso de mídias interativas na primeira infância e desenvolvimento infantil: uma análise multicritério [Quality of interactive media use in early childhood and child development: A multicriteria analysis]. *Jornal de Pediatria, 96*(3), 310–317. https://doi.org/10.1016/j.jped.2018.11.015

Papadopoulou, M. (2016). The "space" of friendship: Young children's understandings and expressions of friendship in a reception class. *Early Child Development and Care, 186*(10), 1544–1558. https://doi.org/10.1080/03004430.2015.1111879

Parent, M., & Rayne, K. (2020). *Human sexuality: A science and story approach*. KendallHunt.

Poulin-Dubois, D., Hastings, P. D., Chiarella, S. S., Geangu, E., Hauf, P., Ruel, A., & Johnson, A. (2018). The eyes know it: Toddlers' visual scanning of sad faces is predicted by their theory of mind skills. *PLOS ONE, 13*(12), Article e0208524. https://doi.org/10.1371/journal.pone.0208524

Pullen Sansfaçon, A., Kirichenko, V., Holmes, C., Feder, S., Lawson, M. L., Ghosh, S., Ducharme, J., Temple Newhook, J., & Suerich-Gulick, F. (2020). Parents' journeys to acceptance and support of gender-diverse and trans children and youth. *Journal of Family Issues, 41*(8), 1214–1236. https://doi.org/10.1177/0192513X19888779

Radesky, J. S., & Christakis, D. A. (2016). Increased screen time: Implications for early childhood development and behavior. *Pediatric Clinics of North America, 63*(5), 827–839. https://doi.org/10.1016/j.pcl.2016.06.006

Ramírez-Villalobos, D., Monterubio-Flores, E., Gonzalez-Vazquez, T. T., Molina-Rodríguez, J. F., Ruelas-González, M. G., & Alcade-Rabanal,

J. E. (2021). Delaying sexual onset: Outcome of a comprehensive sexuality education initiative for adolescents in public schools. *BMC Public Health, 21*(1), Article 1439. https://doi.org/10.1186/s12889-021-11388-2

Rodríguez Fernández, V., & López Ramón y Cajal, C. (2016). *In utero* gratification behaviour in male fetus. *Prenatal Diagnosis, 36*(10), 985–986. https://doi.org/10.1002/pd.4923

Ruba, A. L., & Repacholi, B. M. (2020). Do preverbal infants understand discrete facial expressions of emotion? *Emotion Review, 12*(4), 235–250. https://doi.org/10.1177/1754073919871098

Rudolph, J., & Zimmer-Gembeck, M. J. (2018). Parents as protectors: A qualitative study of parents' views on child sexual abuse prevention. *Child Abuse & Neglect, 85*, 28–38. https://doi.org/10.1016/j.chiabu.2018.08.016

Rudolph, J., Zimmer-Gembeck, M. J., Shanley, D. C., & Hawkins, R. (2018). Child sexual abuse prevention opportunities: Parenting, programs, and the reduction of risk. *Child Maltreatment, 23*(1), 96–106. https://doi.org/10.1177/1077559517729479

Sansfaçon, A. P., Hébert, W., Lee, E. O. J., Faddoul, M., Tourki, D., & Bellot, C. (2018). Digging beneath the surface: Results from stage one of a qualitative analysis of factors influencing the well-being of trans youth in Quebec. *International Journal of Transgenderism, 19*(2), 184–202. https://doi.org/10.1080/15532739.2018.1446066

Schaad, K. A. (2022). Looking for the signs: How childhood narratives define transgender identity. *Sociology Compass, 16*(8), Article e13005. https://doi.org/10.1111/soc4.13005

Sedlak, A. J., Mettenburg, J., Basena, M., Petta, I., McPherson, K., Greene, A., & Li, S. (2010). Executive summary. In *Fourth National Incidence Study of Child Abuse and Neglect (NIS–4): Report to Congress* (pp. 1–22). U.S. Department of Health and Human Services, Administration for Children and Families. https://www.childhelp.org/wp-content/uploads/2015/07/Sedlak-A.-J.-et-al.-2010-Fourth-National-Incidence-Study-of-Child-Abuse-and-Neglect-NIS%E2%80%934.pdf

Shawler, E. B., Elizabeth Bard, M., Taylor, E. K., Wilsie, C., Funderburk, B., & Silovsky, J. F. (2018). Parent–child interaction therapy and young children with problematic sexual behavior: A conceptual overview and treatment considerations. *Children and Youth Services Review, 84*, 206–214. https://doi.org/10.1016/j.childyouth.2017.12.006

Shekhar, S., Maria, A., Kotilahti, K., Huotilainen, M., Heiskala, J. Tuulari, J. J., Hirvi, P., Karlsson, L., Karlsson, H., & Nissilä, I. (2019). Hemodynamic responses to emotional speech in two-month-old infants imaged using diffuse optical tomography. *Scientific Reports, 9*, Article 4745. https://doi.org/10.1038/s41598-019-39993-7

Spiel, E. C., Rodgers, R. F., Paxton, S. J., Wertheim, E. H., Damiano, S. R., Gregg, K. J., & McLean, S. A. (2016). "He's got his father's bias": Parental influence on weight bias in young children. *British Journal of Developmental Psychology, 34*(2), 198–211. https://doi.org/10.1111/bjdp.12123

Spock, B. (1946). *The common sense book of baby and child care.* Duell, Sloan & Pearce.

Spock, B. (2012). *Dr. Spock's baby and child care.* Gallery Books.

Townsend, C., & Rheingold, A. A. (2013, August). *Estimating a child sexual abuse prevalence rate for practitioners: A review of child sexual abuse prevalence studies.* Darkness to Light. https://www.d2l.org/wp-content/uploads/2017/02/PREVALENCE-RATE-WHITE-PAPER-D2L.pdf

Weisgram, E. S., & Dinella, L. M. (Eds.). (2018). *Gender typing of children's toys: How early play experiences impact development.* American Psychological Association. https://doi.org/10.1037/0000077-000

World Health Organization. (1999). *Report of the consultation on child abuse prevention, WHO, Geneva, 29–31 March 1999* (Document No. WHO/HSC/PVI/99.1). https://apps.who.int/iris/handle/10665/65900

Zhao, C., Chronaki, G., Schiessl, I., Wan, M. W., & Abel, K. M. (2019). Is infant neural sensitivity to vocal emotion associated with mother–infant relational experience? *PLOS ONE, 14*(2), Article e0212205. https://doi.org/10.1371/journal.pone.0212205

INDEX

ABOUT THE AUTHORS

Growing up outside Chicago, **Laura Hancock, PhD,** was fascinated by nature, biology, human behavior, and psychology. Consequently, Laura earned her PhD from the University of Texas at Austin in 2009 with a major in biological anthropology and minor in evolutionary psychology. She began teaching sexual health education in 2013 and quickly became one of the few educators to focus on teaching parents about sexuality during early childhood. Laura focuses on providing parents and other caregivers with information about developmentally appropriate sexual behavior and knowledge during the infant, toddler, and kindergarten years. She helps caregivers teach and respond to children in ways that are affirming and lay the foundations of healthy sexuality for a lifetime. Laura resides in Amsterdam, The Netherlands, with her husband and daughter.

Karen Rayne, PhD, has worked in education for the past 2 decades with a specialty in comprehensive sexuality education across the lifespan. She is the cofounder and executive director of UN|HUSHED, where she writes and edits books and lifespan comprehensive sexuality curricula, trains sexuality educators, and builds collaborative coalitions. She is also an assistant professor of instruction at The

University of Texas. Karen has worked with local, national, and international organizations. Her recent books and curricula include *TRANS+: Love, Sex, Romance, and Being You; An Introduction to Sexuality Education: A Handbook for Child Welfare Providers*; and *UN|HUSHED: The Elementary School Curriculum*.